Curing our Ills
The psychology of chronic disease risk, experience and care in Africa

Ama de-Graft Aikins

BSc (Manchester), MSc (Manchester Met), PhD (London)
Professor of Social Psychology
Regional Institute for Population Studies, University of Ghana, Legon

Inaugural Lecture delivered at the Great Hall, University of Ghana,
on 30th June 2016

First published in Ghana 2018 for
THE UNIVERSITY OF GHANA by
Sub-Saharan Publishers
P.O.Box 358
Legon-Accra
Ghana
Email: saharanp@africaonline.com.gh
Website: www.subsaharanpublishers.com

Regional Institute for Population Studies
University of Ghana
P.O.Box LG 96
Legon - Accra
Ghana
Tel: +233-302-50074
website: http://www.ug.edu.gh

ISBN: 978-9988-8830-2-7

Cover image: Asante Adinkra symbol of life transformation titled
Sesa wo suban, which means 'change or transform your character' or
'change or transform your life'.

Contents

Figures

FOREWORD

Inaugural lectures at University of Ghana have always been memorable events that allow the academic community to appreciate the scope of a researcher's work over a period. They are expected to inform the world about a researcher's contribution to their discipline and to the generation of new knowledge in general. They are usually met with great expectation. These lectures have usually been published by the University as one of its main public documents.

In June 2016, Professor Ama de-Graft Aikins delivered her Inaugural Lecture at the Great Hall of the University. She spoke on the theme "Curing our ills: the psychology of chronic disease risk, experience and care in Africa". I was in the Chair. It was indeed a memorable occasion for me as it was one of the last few Inaugural Lectures that I chaired before stepping down as Vice Chancellor. It was very well delivered and was well received by the large audience that attended the event. For many people the lecture focused on a topic that they could easily appreciate in view of the growing relevance of chronic conditions to the Ghanaian population.

The lecture covered a wide range of issues on the risk, management and care of chronic diseases from a psychological perspective. It began with an introduction to the kind of psychology that Professor de-Graft Aikins is interested in and is associated with: the sub-field of critical social psychology. The second part of the lecture focused on "The psychology of chronic disease risk, experiences and care". She discussed the complex context of chronic disease risk, problems associated with living with diabetes including the psychological struggles that come with it, and care in family and healthcare settings. In the final part, titled "Curing our ills", Professor de-Graft Aikins turned her attention to finding solutions to the myriad of problems that people with chronic diseases, especially diabetes, face.

It is important to recognize the fact that this inaugural lecture dealt with one of the fastest growing challenges of health systems in Africa. While global health discourse has tended to prioritise infectious diseases for obvious reasons, there is growing evidence that chronic non-communicable diseases (NCDs) are becoming a major force to reckon with in most parts of the region. Many of these conditions are associated with lifestyle changes that have taken place in the last few decades, which are generally linked to globalization and rapid urbanisation. Professor de-Graft Aikins's research belongs to a growing cohort of important NCD research on Africans at home and abroad by multidisciplinary researchers. It is a field that some African universities, including University of Ghana, are beginning to devote considerable resources. Through this work our understanding of how the diseases affect men and women, and how they can be managed, is also improving. We can only thank these researchers who are devoting time and resources to help us develop interventions that will lead to better management of different chronic diseases.

Ernest Aryeetey
Vice Chancellor (2010-2016)
University of Ghana

INTRODUCTION

Vice Chancellor, Pro Vice Chancellors, Registrar, Provosts, Deans, Directors, Former Vice Chancellors, Distinguished Ladies and Gentlemen, I am grateful for the opportunity to deliver my inaugural lecture this evening.

In this Great Hall, I am sure some of us have heard about or know someone with diabetes or hypertension, a second set of us is caring for a loved one with either condition and a third set of us lives with either condition or both. Within the first two sets, at least 50% of us aged 30 and above are likely to have high blood pressure or impaired glucose tolerance and not know it. Hypertension, diabetes and other chronic diseases like stroke and cancers have become major causes of disability and premature death for millions of Ghanaians and Africans. In 2005, the World Health Organization (WHO), observed that prevalence rates of chronic non-communicable diseases (NCDs) were highest in Africa and predicted that Africa would have the fastest rate of prevalence, morbidity and mortality in the coming decades. This prediction has come true. Chronic conditions are lifelong and incurable, they require long-term treatment and management which can be expensive, and they often lead to complex complications and additional conditions which undermine the quality of life of affected individuals and their families. The WHO, along with other global health organizations, rightly emphasise that we need to address this public health challenge urgently because of its impact on individuals, families, communities, health systems and governments.

In this lecture I will discuss the psychology of chronic disease risk, experience and care in Africa. In a brief Part 1, I will describe the kind of psychology I do, to set the context for the lecture. In part 2, I will focus on the second half of my title. I will talk about: the psychology of risk; the psychology of experience; and the psychology of care. I will focus on diabetes and will show why diabetes is a theoretically significant condition for this discussion. I will also draw attention to why we need a critical psychological analysis of these themes. In part 3, I will synthesise the evidence by returning to the first half of my title: 'curing our ills'. I treat 'ills' in terms of the physical as well as the ideological. I conceptualise ideological ills as the ways health experts - researchers, practitioners, policymakers, funders and development partners - define our problems and develop solutions to our problems, thereby setting the broader structural framework in which we manage our daily lives, in health, in illness, and increasingly, in dying. I argue that the physical and ideological ills are interconnected and, as a result, must be addressed through interdisciplinary approaches. To conclude, I will offer practical solutions for reducing chronic disease risk and improving the quality of long-term experience and care.

For all these stages, I will refer to a synthesised body of psychological, health and social science knowledge generated on the themes. This will include my independent and collaborative work, carried out over the last 16 years, on: diabetes experiences in Ghana, diabetes experiences among Ghanaian migrants in Europe, mental health in Ghana, health systems in Ghana, health systems responses to the NCD burden in Ghana and Africa and low and middle income countries, and the role of psychology in addressing health and social problems affecting African communities[1].

---

1   On diabetes experiences in Ghana see de-Graft Aikins, 2003, 2004, 2005a, 2006; de-Graft Aikins et al 2012, 2014a, 2014b; on diabetes experiences among Ghanaian migrants in Europe see Agyemang et al 2014, 2016; on mental health in Ghana see de-Graft Aikins and Ofori-Atta, 2007; de-Graft Aikins, 2015; on health systems in Ghana see de-Graft Aikins and Koram, 2017; on health systems responses to the NCD burden in Ghana and Africa and in low and middle income countries see de-Graft Aikins et al, 2010a, 2010b, 2012, 2013, 2016; de-Graft Aikins and Agyemang, 2017; and on the role of psychology in addressing health and social problems affecting African communities see de-Graft Aikins and Marks, 2007; de-Graft Aikins, 2012, 2014; de-Graft Aikins et al, 2014c, 2015.

My work has involved interviewing, having situated conversations and observing over 1000 Ghanaians across the country in all regions, but Western region, and Ghanaians living in three European countries (UK, Netherlands and Germany[2]).

My main collaborators have been Professor Francis Dodoo, Professor Kwadwo Koram and Dr Barima Afranie at Legon, Professor Charles Agyemang at the University of Amsterdam, Professor Gbenga Ogedegbe at New York University, Dr Juliet Addo at London School of Hygiene and Tropical Medicine, and Professor Ernestina Coast at the London School of Economics and Political Science (LSE).

This body of work has also formed the basis for PhD training at my institute, the Regional Institute for Population Studies (RIPS). I have 5 PhD students working on various aspects of population health and NCDs with whom I have discussed and developed new directions in research - and who also helped me with last minute data collection and analysis for this lecture - and I must acknowledge them. They are: Tobi Sanuade, Sandra Boatemaa, Raphael Baffour Awuah, Mawuli Kushitor and Ernest Afrifa-Anane[3].

Over the last 10 years my understanding of chronic illness experience in Ghana – for sufferers and caregivers - has deepened as I became a primary caregiver of my father and my mother. My father had hypertension and suffered multiple strokes over a nine-year period, each more debilitating than the previous: he passed away in November 2014. My mother lives with diabetes and hypertension. I sought permission from my mother to make use of specific insights from my family experience in highlighting some of the complex dynamics of chronic illness experience and care in Part Two of the lecture.

---

2   See Appendix 1 for an overview of my research projects and locations.

3   All five have since completed their PhDs successfully.

Finally, I have been involved in NCD policy development, and health systems research, at the national and international levels. Major opportunities I have had in this area have come as a result of the support of two mentors: Professor David Ofori-Adjei (former Director of Noguchi Memorial Institute for Medical Research, Legon and former Rector of the Ghana College of Physicians and Surgeons) and the late Dr Sam Adjei (former Deputy Director General of the Ghana Health Service). In part 3, I will draw on the lessons I have learned from the health policy and global health spaces to address the challenges relating to our ideological ills.

PART 1: CRITICAL SOCIAL PSYCHOLOGY

Definitions and sub-fields of Psychology

When I decided to switch paths from an undergraduate degree in pharmacology to graduate training in psychology, I kept getting asked: what can you do with psychology in Ghana? This was in 1996. Twenty years on, there is greater awareness about psychology in Ghana. Because now, whenever I am asked what I do and I say I am a psychologist, the response invariably is: "so can you tell me what I am thinking?" I escape by saying I am off mindreading duty. While it is great to be perceived to have the superpower of mind reading, Psychology is not that exact a science or art. It is also much more complex than that.

The common textbook definition states that psychology is the science of mental life, the science of mind and behaviour, and variations on these themes. These definitions boil down to a focus on how *people think, feel and act*. However, depending on where one was trained and which branch (or sub-field) of psychology one belongs to, the approach to examining how people think, feel and act will be different. There are at least 20 different branches in psychology, including established branches like developmental psychology and newer ones like environmental psychology. In Ghana, ten sub-fields of psychology are taught or practised in six institutions (see Figure 1).

Within the broad branches, theorists and practitioners take a philosophical approach, a positivistic (or hard science) approach or a critical science approach. These differences have arisen from the "various scientific revolutions", to quote Thomas Kuhn (1962), that have occurred in the global discipline throughout its long history.

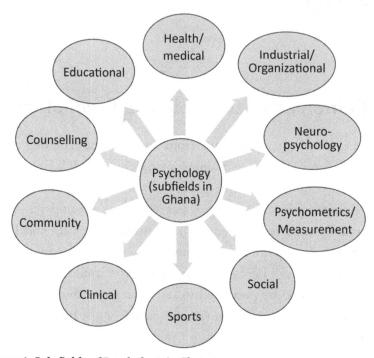

Figure 1. Sub-fields of Psychology in Ghana

Sources: de-Graft Aikins et al, 2014; Akotia and Mate-Kole, 2014. Universities with Psychology
           Programmes: University of Ghana ; University of Cape Coast; University of Education,
           Winneba; Methodist University; Central University; Trinity Theological Seminary.

So, there have been revolutions around the nature of how
people think, feel and act: the technical stuff of psychology. We
have had trends including Sigmund Freud's psychoanalysis (which
examines the psyche as the engine that drives behaviour), B.F.
Skinner's behaviourism (which privileges observable behaviour over
the workings of the mind) and Carl Rogers' humanistic psychology
(which privileges the lived experience of the whole person).

Within these revolutions, there have been debates about
whether people think, feel and act in the same way everywhere in
the world: "the universal vs particular" conundrum. For example,
is intelligence universal or particular? The universalist group argue
that intelligence is universal, therefore IQ tests developed in the US

among college students can be applied to Ghanaian rural farmers without formal education. The particularists argue that intelligence is context specific, that each culture has its own 'folk psychology', so tests have to be developed or validated within target cultures or research communities.[4]

The critical turn in Psychology

In the late 1960s through early 1970s, an ideological movement occurred in psychology, called the 'critical turn'. This event in psychology was spearheaded by European and Latin American psychologists, and was part of a broader 'critical turn' in the social sciences and humanities.

What inspired the critical turn in psychology, were three issues[5]. First, the dominant mainstream psychology lacked social relevance: it was not speaking to the major social and political shifts of the day such as the civil rights movement in America or the decolonization struggles in Africa. Secondly, it focused on parochial problems but

---

4   The universalist view has spawned a large body of research on race, ethnicity and intelligence which associates differences in intelligence to racial and ethnic differences, rather than environmental factors. This field buys into the 'scientific racism' of the colonial era where psychological and psychiatric research sought to prove the superiority of western cultures and the inferiority of African cultures and peoples. Scientific racism generates controversial views from prominent and obscure scientists alike, such as that from James Watson, winner of a Nobel prize for genetics (for his work with Francis Crick on the DNA). Watson aired his view that Africans were less intelligent than Westerners when he asserted: "All our social policies are based on the fact that their intelligence is the same as ours - whereas all the testing says not really". Such views were robustly challenged during the colonial era and continue to be challenged today. The particularist view is aligned with context-situated analysis and interpretation. For example Christopher and colleagues observe: "Every society has a folk psychology consisting of characteristic ways of construing development, personality, group relations, psychological disturbances, and so on" (Christopher et al, 2014). See Richards (1997) on the history of race and racism in Psychology, especially in relation to research in Africa.

5   See Burton and Kagan, 2005.

projected these problems as universally valid (the earlier example I gave on intelligence testing). Finally, it imitated the scientific neutrality of the physical sciences which meant it ignored the moral dimension of social scientific phenomena.

What critical psychologists sought to do was to address the deficiencies in the dominant system, by explicitly examining the social, cultural, economic and political contexts of psychological life.

I was trained in the critical social psychological tradition at the doctoral and postdoctoral levels. This tradition sees social psychology as a bridge science that integrates "psychology, sociology and cultural anthropology into an instrument for studying group life"[6]. At the London School of Economics and Political Science (LSE) and Cambridge, where I was trained, I joined a research group whose work was informed by the Theory of Social Representations, a social psychological theory developed by the French theorist Serge Moscovici in the 1950s.

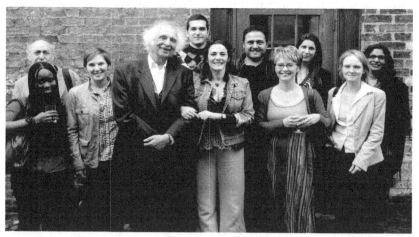

The LSE-Cambridge Social Representations Theory (SRT) Group

Serge Moscovici (front row, third from left), with members of the SRT group during a meeting held at Cambridge in 2005; in the group are the late Cambridge academic Gerard Duveen (back row, left); LSE professor of social psychology Sandra Jovchelovitch (front row, fourth from left, arms locked with Moscovici); and Ama de-Graft Aikins (front row, left).

---

6   Moscovici and Markova, 2006, p.39

The Theory of Social Representations

Social representations are defined, within Social Representations Theory (hereafter SRT), as practical everyday social knowledge that is produced, shared, used and transformed in social life[7]. Theorists emphasise that social representations are produced by 'competing versions of reality': everyday knowledge has elements of consensus, conflict and absence because social groups - the producers of social knowledge - are heterogeneous. Social representations also 'create reality': the process of producing everyday knowledge creates new meanings and social identities that are projected into the social world.

SRT aims to "conceptualise, simultaneously, both the power of society and the agency of individuals"[8]. There is general agreement that social psychological processes operate at mutually influential levels linking individual level processes to societal level processes. These psychological processes are often related at different levels of social organization, but each level has a unique structure and associated meanings. Serge Moscovici (1988, p. 288), for instance, argues:

> "There is a world of difference between representations envisaged at the person to person level and the level of relations between individuals and group, or at the level of a society's common consciousness. At each level, representations have a completely different meaning. The phenomena are related but different."

In Figure 2, I show the four levels of analysis offered by the Swiss social psychologist, Willem Doise[9]. The 'psychological' or 'intrapersonal' level, focuses on how the individual interprets the

---

7   Moscovici and Duveen, 2000; Rose et al, 1995

8   Gervais et al, 1999, p.422

9   Doise, 1986

world; the 'interpersonal' level, focuses on the character of the interaction between individuals considered as interchangeable partners in a situation; the 'positional' level, considers the different social positions of actors in situational interactions; and the 'ideological' level, focuses on broader belief systems.

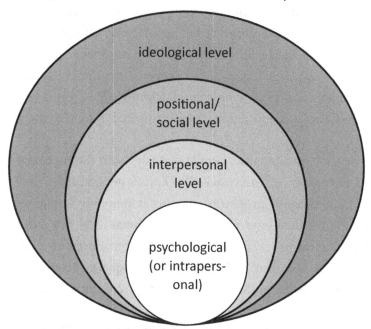

Figure 2. Levels of Analysis in Social Psychology

Let's take love in a young Ghanaian Christian's life (see Figure 3). A girl, let's call her Akua, falls in love (this is the psychological or intrapersonal level). Her love interest is a boy in church, Kwame, who loves her back but probably not with the same motivations (that's the interpersonal level). Akua and Kwame are youth choiristers and their fellow members will tease them about their relationship, suggesting that 'being in love' is acceptable (the positional or social level). However, Christian and their church doctrine instructs that, unlike worldly unbelievers, they cannot fully consummate their love until they get married (that is the ideological or belief system level). At each level love is similar but different. The moment these lovebirds contemplate rebelling against church doctrine, is the point at which the 'power of society' and the 'agency of individuals' meet. Of course individual agency has positive and negative outcomes, which will also be manifested at our four levels of analyses. I will come back to Akua and Kwame again.

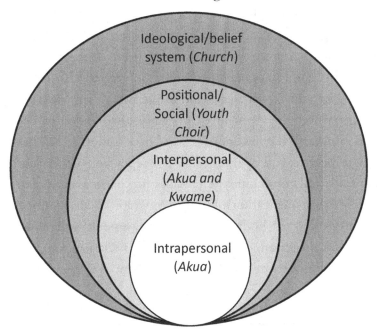

Figure 3. Love at four levels of social psychological analysis

Ideally, researchers should understand how a social psychological phenomenon, like love, operates at or across different levels of analysis. There are a number of technical instructions that go with this that I won't bore you all with[10]. But essentially what this means

---

10   Willem Doise (1986) notes, an applied social psychology "requires enrichment of a given theoretical model by other models so as to construct a more complete approach to reality by reduction of the unexplained in each model" (p.26)". Michael Murray (2000), discussing the importance of levels of analysis in health psychology, advocates bringing together a number of conceptual perspectives, including Doise's, on understanding the illness experience. Murray (2000) observes that "for a critical health psychology the challenge is to move beyond the dominant personal

is that critical psychologists are free to borrow appropriate concepts from within psychology and outside of psychology if this helps us develop critical analysis of our subject matter at our chosen levels of analysis.

My PhD thesis examined social representations of diabetes in Ghana and was grounded in a critical synthesis of concepts and empirical insights from health psychology, the sociology of health, and anthropology of health and illness in African communities[11]. Much of the work I have done since has been conceptualised through the SRT lens. I have been particularly interested in a central concept called cognitive polyphasia and in the role of emotions in everyday experience (see Appendix 2). I have also tended to use SRT within a broader framework of critical psychology, which has allowed me to borrow and operationalise concepts from other sub-fields like health and community psychology (e.g participation) and other disciplines like medical sociology (e.g biographical disruption), medical anthropology (e.g body-self, explanatory models) and public health (e.g political economy of global health)[12]. I will use some of these concepts in my lecture and I will define them as they appear.

---

level of analysis to consider more social processes" (p.345). In Julie Hepworth's (2004) discussion of the sub-field of public health psychology she observes that the "the application of psychology [to public health] needs to extend across all levels of population health; individual, social, structural and environmental" (p.46). Hepworth further argues: "A single theory simply cannot establish an integrative approach within a field such as public health that is premised on multiplicity... neither is it desirable to reduce the integrative framework of public health and psychology to a single theory." (p 46).

11   de-Graft Aikins, A (2005). *Social representations of diabetes in Ghana: recon-structing self, society and culture.* Unpublished PhD Thesis, London School of Economics and Political Science.

12   See Campbell and Jovchelovitch (2000) on participation; Bury (1982) on biographi-cal disruption; Scheper-Hughes and Locke (1987) and Helman(2000) on body-self; Kleinman (1980) on explanatory models; Clarke (2014) on the political economy of global health.

PART 2: THE PSYCHOLOGY OF CHRONIC DISEASE RISK, EXPERIENCES AND CARE

The Psychology of Chronic Disease Risk

The major chronic conditions that affect Ghanaians and Africans are hypertension, stroke, diabetes, cancers and chronic respiratory diseases[13]. Other common chronic conditions include mental health disorders like depression and anxiety, those affecting children, like sickle cell disease, and those affecting the elderly like arthritis and dementia.

Because of the long term and costly nature of the major chronic diseases, prevention is key and this requires an understanding of our risk status and how we manage our risk status. According to global health scientists the five dominant NCDs are linked by four major risk factors: unhealthy eating, physical inactivity, harmful use of alcohol and smoking[14]. These factors are collectively called modifiable risk factors, because we can control them. There are also non-modifiable risks that we cannot control: like our sex, our age, and our genetics. For instance I am a high risk candidate for hypertension and diabetes because my father had hypertension and mother lives with both conditions.

---

13   The African continent has the highest prevalence of hypertension at 46%. Hypertension is a well-established precursor to heart attacks and stroke. In Ghana, prevalence of hypertension is between 25% and 48%, with higher rates in urban areas. Type 2 diabetes prevalence ranges between 6% in Accra and 9% in Kumasi; rates of 12% have been recorded among civil servants in Accra.

14   Some researchers add psychosocial stress to the list, although this has not been subjected to rigorous research (see Agyemang et al, 2009). See Appendix 3 for notes on the modifiable risk factors and WHO endorsed strategies for addressing these risk factors and prevention the associated NCDs.

The modifiable risk factors are usually attributed to lifestyle, with the implicit sense that we choose to eat badly, not to engage in physical activity, drink alcohol to harmful levels, and smoke tobacco, because we want to, or because we have developed habits or our social circumstances lead us to behave in these ways. Some researchers refer to NCD risk being transmitted socially through "peer effects", such as when young people pressure friends to smoke, or middle aged African women normalise fatness[15].

There is a broader argument in the critical health sciences – e.g. public health, health policy, sociology and health psychology - that we must understand risk also in terms of structural forces, such as the 'political economy of global public health'[16]. Political economy refers to 'the mutually reinforcing interplay between politics and economics at the structural level'.[17]

I will use food as an example to explain this concept further. Obesity rates among Ghanaian women have tripled over the last 20 years, from 4.7% in 1993 to 15.3% in 2014[18]. Male rates are reported to be far lower than the female rates. Overweight/obesity occurs when we consume high energy foods and do not expend the energy through physical activity, for example. How did we get to this stage?

---

15   Surcke et al, 2006, p.33. observe: "recently, a small but growing amount of research has pointed out that while biological transmission usually does not occur for non-communicable diseases, risk factors may well be transmitted socially. In particular, it has been shown that peers (broadly defined as classmates, friends, siblings, even to some extent parents) influence people's health behaviour. The evidence of 'peer effects' appears strongest in the case of adolescent substance abuse, but evidence has also emerged in the area of diet and physical activity"

16   Hepworth, 2004; Clarke, 2014.

17   Sackrey et al (2013, pp 3-4, citing Riddell et al, 2009) offer this definition of political economy: "Political economy…is more concerned [than mainstream economics] with the relationships of the economic system and its institutions to the rest of society and social development. It is sensitive to the influence of non-economic factors such as political and social institutions, morality and ideology in determining economic events. It thus has a *much broader focus* than [mainstream] economics"

18   Abubakari et al, 2008; Agyemang et al, 2016

The simple 'lifestyle' argument will say our taste buds have changed, we crave new foods, and the more westernised the better. And because these processes have occurred over a long period of time, this would seem intuitively true to us.

In some communities in Accra and Cape Coast processed foods were common in the colonial era[19]. By the 1930s, according to Legon historian Professor Irene Odotei, the dietary habits of Osu had westernised to such a degree that a popular Ga saying was: '*Osu borla, sardine chinsi so*'[20]. By the 1960s newly independent Ghanaians had become so accustomed (or shall we say deeply addicted) to processed foods like sugar, milk, corned beef and sardines, that part of the reason Nkrumah was overthrown was because the country had run out of these *"essential commodities"*[21].

Ghanaians aged over 40 will remember that in the 1970s and 1980s jollof rice with chicken and gem biscuits were only consumed at Christmas, and one had to journey to upmarket hotels like Ambassador hotel (now the Movenpick) to have burgers and club sandwiches[22]. 'Minerals' were rationed even in middle class homes[23]. Now these foods and drinks are consumed everyday[24].

---

19   Field, 1939; Quayson, 2014; Robertson, 1984.

20   Loosely translated as, the rubbish heaps of Osu are full of sardine tins

21   When older Ghanaians speak of the period, they recall long queues of people waiting outside stores to buy fast diminishing supplies of 'essenco'. The deep importance afforded to essential commodities by Ghanaians was underscored by the conferment of a popular nickname: 'essenco'.

22   Jollof rice – a popular Ghanaian and West African dish made of rice cooked in tomato sauce, chilli and spices, and for some cooks, meat and fish. Mode of preparation similar to the Spanish paella or the Louisiana Creole jambalaya. Gem biscuits were produced by Picadilly Biscuits Limited, which was established in Ghana in the 1960s.

23   In Ghana, 'minerals' refer to locally bottled coke, sprite, fanta and other fizzy drinks. The term extends to imported canned versions and newer plastic bottle versions.

24   Agyei-Mensah and de-Graft Aikins (2010, p. 890) observe: "Today, fast-food places range from services modeled on Papaye to international franchises such as

The difference today, which brings in the element of political economy, is that our changing taste buds have aligned with a system of food market globalization. 50 years after the long queues that led to Nkrumah's overthrow, Ghana now has an abundance of 'essential commodities'. In preparation for this lecture my team did a quick survey of 3 supermarkets: All Needs on Legon campus, Max Mart in East Legon and Blessed Assurance in Ga Mashie. We found 22 different brands of rice, 30 brands of oil, 13 brands of sugar, 17 brands of milk, 10 brands of corned beef, 18 brands of sardines; 43 brands of juices and 15 brands of energy drinks (see Figure 4). Some brands had as many as 10 variations of the same product.

We see, then, that the rising rates of overweight and obesity are not due solely to changing cultural tastes and free will. Overweight and obesity rates are also increasing because of the sheer abundance of unhealthy food commodities on our streets and in our markets and shops. Food markets have become more globalized, such that commodities that originated from one source, or two, decades ago (e.g two foreign brands of sugar, St Louis and Tate & Lyle, in 1960) now originate from several sources (e.g 13 foreign and local brands of sugar from 13 manufacturers in 2016).

Nandos and Bonjour (On the Run). These restaurants are usually located in wealthy neighborhoods, shopping districts and malls, and at gas stations, and they tend to serve up-market clientele. Cheaper kiosk versions of fast food—termed check check—usually located within markets, truck stations, and along Accra's busy roads, make brisk business with the less wealthy. American style fast-food restaurants coexist with restaurants serving affordable, traditional Ghanaian meals to a growing workforce that lives too far away in Accra's outlying suburbs to eat lunch at home. Both American-style fastfoods and Ghanaian traditional meals can be unhealthy, with high levels of sugar, salt and saturated fats, often consumed with high sugar content sodas, or "minerals"."

22 brands of rice	30 brands of oil	13 brands of sugar
Aoun; Babrina; Belle France; Casa Rinaldi; China Rice; Cindy; Divella; Ewoe; Fortune; Gino; India Gate; Lele; Millicent; My Dear; Natco; Royal Aroma; Royal Feast; Ruby; Sultana; Uncle Ben; Uncle Sam; Waitrose.	Agnior; Best In; Blue Dragon; Borges; Casa Pinaldi; Casa Rinaldi; Crisco; Crisp and Dry; Divella; Essential Waitrose/Waitrose; Filippo Berio; Flora; Frytol; Gino; Golden Plate; Granivita; Homefoods; Lee Kum Kee; Levo; Mazola; Napolina; Obaapa; Roda; Roder; Serafina; Sole Mio; Unoli; Viking; Wesson; Zea;	2000; Argentina white sugar; Brazilian white sugar; Comperchee; Crystal; Fair Trade; Khater; Max mart store brand; Silverspoon; St Louis; Sugar Daddy; Sunny; Tate &Lyle.

17 brands of milk	10 brands of corned beef	18 brands of sardines
Carnation; Cowbell; Dano; Dayson; Emborg; Essential Waitrose; Even; Ideal; Incolac; Lele; Marvel; Miksi; Milky; Nido; Nuno; Peak; President;	Altaghziah; Bella; Ester ; Exeter; Festival; Geisha; Grace; Heinz; Lele; Obaapa; Princes; Rambo	African Queen; Bella; Belma; Best In; Ena Pa; Essential Waitrose; Ester; Geisha; John West; Lele; Milo; Mother; Obaapa; Princes; Princess; Smile; Tinio; Titus;

43 brands of juice	15 brands of energy drinks
Aloe Fresh; BB; Bella; Belle France; Best In; Boijos; Bonita; Capri Sun; Ceres; Character; Cheers; Chinchin; Colypso; Dada; DJ; Don Simon; Elisha; Essential Waitrose; Fan Dango; Freeze; Frutelli; Fusli; Grand Juicy; Juicy; Just Juice; Kalyppo; Maccaw; Magic Bar; Magiclicious; Magic Time; Ocean Spray; Prestige; Pure Heaven; Pure Joy; Ribena; Sampellecrino; So Fresh; Squiz; Stute; Tampico; Top Up; U Fresh; Villa Vita	Atonne; Best In; Blue Jeans; Hype; Lucozade; Magic; Powerhouse; Powerplay; Purdeys; Rash; Red Bull; Rox; Rush; Storm; Vicco;

Figure 4. 'Essential Commodities' in three neighbourhood shops in Accra, June 2016

These seismic changes have been backed by aggressive advertising strategies. So, we have billboards advertising, without irony, the 'heart healthy' qualities of coke (a soda that has between 12 and 16 teaspoons of sugar, depending on where the product is manufactured) and the health benefits of processed white perfumed rice (a product that has been stripped of its basic micronutrients).

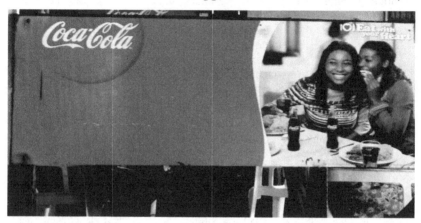

"Eat with your heart" Coca-Cola advert at various urban Ghanaian locations

Crucially, the government plays an enabling role. The rising overweight/obesity rates can also be attributed to how successive Ghanaian governments have made poor choices about regulating importation of commodities and supporting local agricultural industries. It is reported that sugar was the fourth largest import in Ghana, after rice, fish and poultry; and the NDC government spent $400million importing sugar each year.

Since its inauguration on Accra's Oxford Street in 2012, KFC has expanded its reach in Accra and beyond, unchecked, as part of its project of global domination in Africa, Latin America and Asia.

Given this complex context of food abundance and choice, it is not surprising that there has been an exponential expansion of Ghanaian waistlines over the last 20 years. The impact of food market globalization on food habits and overweight and obesity is reported for other African countries[25].

Similar political economy arguments can be made about the other modifiable lifestyle risk factors of NCDs in particular alcohol overconsumption, where an aggressive bitters industry aligns with the complex psychology of male virility.

To summarise, health scientists define NCD risk in terms of non-modifiable biological factors (sex, age, genetics), modifiable social factors (lifestyle: individual and social habits) and structural factors (economic, political). I will refer to these definitions as *'scientific logic'*: that is knowledge developed by the health sciences community that draws on empirical evidence from various relevant disciplines, including medicine, epidemiology, public health and health economics.

So how do lay Africans and Ghanaians define and manage NCD risk?

How lay Ghanaians and Africans define NCD Risk

Early research on African health beliefs and practices, proposed that Africans drew on a tripartite system in making sense of illness. The system had three elements: natural, social and supernatural (see figure 5)[26].

Naturally caused conditions occurred through natural elements such as heat, cold, injuries and pollution, and included malaria, fevers and general aches and pains. Socially caused conditions occurred through 'conscious or unconscious interpersonal malevolence'[27]

---

25   Abubakari et al, 2008; Agyemang et al, 2016

26   The Ghanaian sociologist, Patrick A. Twumasi in his book *'Traditional Medical Systems of Ghana'* refers to spiritually caused conditions (*Sunsum mu yadee*), physically caused conditions (*ho nam mu yadee*) and economically or socially oriented conditions (*asetana mu asem*) (Twumasi, 1975)

27   Helman, 2000, p.93.

and were sub-classified under witchcraft and sorcery, now popularly known as 'African electronics'[28]. Supernaturally caused conditions were caused through the direct action of supernatural beings such as gods and ancestral spirits. Rare or unnatural events such as the death of a child or young adult, chronic illnesses or illnesses which caused sudden death in otherwise healthy adults were attributed to social or supernatural forces. While the origins of these conditions were perceived to be serious and mysterious, people believed that some were ultimately curable. Theorists argued that treatment seeking behaviour was influenced by these causal theories of illness. If an individual attributed their condition to natural causes, they were more likely to seek treatment within biomedical systems, which were viewed as experts in treating physical conditions. If the attribution was to the spiritual or supernatural, they would seek treatment with systems with expertise in spiritual and supernatural interventions, such as shrine priests.

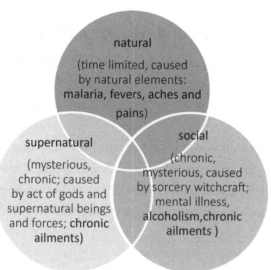

Figure 5. The tripartite model of disease attributions in Africa

28   McCool, 2015

Some of these early findings are still relevant today. But the current evidence is more nuanced. From my work on social representations of diabetes, two key insights emerge. First, individuals make sense of chronic conditions in very complex ways that blend the boundaries between natural, social and supernatural explanations, and move beyond these three categories[29]. Second, causal attributions do not lead to treatment seeking behaviours in the predictable and linear manner proposed by the tripartite model.

The content and sources of diabetes knowledge are complex. Lay individuals attribute diabetes to natural factors (heredity, ageing, and gender), social factors (poor lifestyles including poor diets, lack of physical activity and alcohol overconsumption, psychosocial stress), supernatural factors (witchcraft, sorcery) and structural factors (poverty, contaminated food staples produced by toxic agricultural practices) (see Figure 6).

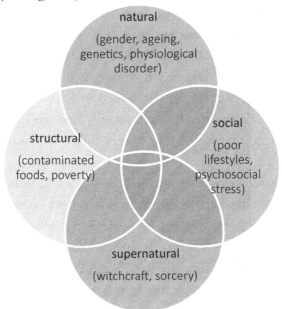

Figure 6. Lay causal theories of diabetes in Ghana

29   de-Graft Aikins, 2004, 2005b, 2006; de-Graft Aikins et al, 2014

Individuals do not only draw on multiple causal theories (e.g sugar, sorcery and poverty), they also speak of diabetes in ways that suggest the theories are intricately intertwined. A natural causal theory can have supernatural roots: for instance the heritable nature of diabetes can be driven by witchcraft (see the story of Maame and Akosua in Appendix 4). Also, individuals receive information from unexpected sources. For example spiritual causal theories are not only expounded by herbalists and shrine priests in diagnostic encounters; they are also proffered by health workers in hospitals and community health centres (see Afia's story in Appendix 4).

The functions of diabetes knowledge are also complex. For example attributing diabetes to witchcraft or sorcery, does not necessarily lead to treatment seeking with shrine priests or charismatic Christian faith healers. Focusing on experiences of diabetes, the familial context of caregiving and the social context of perceptions and social relations, reveal how knowledge, intentions and everyday illness actions are shaped by complex social factors such as financial status, geographical access to medical treatment, access to alternative diets, social support and stigma. Treatment-seeking behaviour is therefore influenced by illness causal theories *as well as* other factors such as the severity and timeframe of the illness and the cost, availability, and accessibility of pluralistic health services[30].

This Ghanaian evidence is mirrored across African countries where similar studies on diabetes attributions have been conducted, including Cameroon, Botswana, Tanzania and Zimbabwe.[31]

So, like global health scientists, lay people have natural, social, and structural explanations for NCDs. But lay people also draw on supernatural causal theories. Furthermore, while aspects of

---

30   de-Graft Aikins, 2005

31   Awah et al, 2008a, 2008b; Hjelm and Mufunda, 2010; Kolling et al, 2010; Sabone, 2008.

their knowledge are drawn from professional biomedical sources, their wider eclectic knowledge base is informed by a range of sources beyond biomedicine: family, friends, community networks, pluralistic healthcare providers, and increasingly, the mass media. Their attribution process is what SRT theorists will call 'cognitive polyphasic' (see Appendix 2). The result is social logic: an expanded repertoire of lay NCD knowledge that draws on health sciences (however well or poorly understood), but moves beyond this to socio-cultural sources, including common sense, religion, and politics.

How lay Ghanaians and Africans Manage NCD Risk

Despite growing awareness of the rising levels of NCDs across the continent, risk perceptions are poor. There is an understanding of the underlying risk factors, especially of diet and overweight/obesity. However while people know that NCDs are a problem they do not believe that they themselves are at risk. In Ghana, up to 70% of people who are screened as having hypertension, in various screening exercises, do not know they are hypertensive[32].

Health psychologists have shown that the relationships between awareness, knowledge, intention and behaviour are complex and unpredictable. Awareness of a problem and understanding of the problem are important but are not enough to change behaviour. For example, in Ghana there is near universal HIV awareness and knowledge of risk factors; yet condom use is low (2%) and abortion prevalence is high (7.1%). Both sets of statistics suggest that individuals are having unsafe sex.

Psychologists also argue that the symbolic and material circumstances of everyday life shape the knowledge-attitude-

---

32   Bosu, 2012; Awuah et al, 2014; Addo et al, 2012

behaviour relation. Not having enough time or money for instance, can thwart an individual's best intentions to eat properly or have a medical check-up. Secondly even when people know they might be at risk of NCDs they might process this through the lens of 'hierarchies of risk'[33]. This involves weighing options of what presents the greatest risk to one's health and life and dealing with that. This is why a poor mother with breast cancer or uncontrolled diabetes in Accra or Dar-es-Salaam, will prioritise their child's nutritional and health needs over their own pressing needs[34].

To summarise, three insights emerge on the psychology of risk. First, there is greater overlap between social logic and scientific logic than we give lay people credit for. By extension, we must be aware that diagnostic and treatment practices of healthcare professionals can also be informed by a blend of scientific and social logic. Second, awareness and knowledge of NCDs are not enough to change risky health behaviours; one must understand the complex mediating role of everyday life and competing priorities. Finally, within the context of disabling environments, such as that caused by food market globalization, some preventive health behaviours are difficult to adopt.

This complex social, cultural and economic context of population risk creates the conditions for the rising numbers of people with chronic conditions.

---

33   Crossley, 2000

34   Dedey et al, 2016; Kolling et al, 2010

The Psychology of Chronic Disease Experience

Critical health scientists distinguish between disease and illness. Disease refers to the biomedical emphasis on organic pathology and illness refers to the subjective experience of pain and disability[35].

Diabetes is defined as a "chronic disease that occurs either when the pancreas does not produce enough insulin - a hormone that regulates blood sugar - or when the body cannot effectively use the insulin it produces"[36]. There are two main types. Type 1 diabetes (also known as insulin-dependent, juvenile or childhood-onset) occurs when insulin production is deficient and requires daily insulin treatment. Type 2 diabetes (also known as non-insulin-dependent, or adult-onset) occurs when the body is unable to use insulin effectively. Globally, the majority of people live with type 2 diabetes: and this has been the focus of my research with Ghanaians[37]. Insulin deficiencies and irregularities result in raised levels of blood glucose, which can damage many bodily systems, but most crucially blood vessels and nerves. Raised blood-glucose levels can lead to a range of acute and chronic medical complications. The acute complications include hyperglycaemia (very high blood sugar) and hypoglycaemia (very low blood sugar). The chronic complications include blindness and foot complications. The effects of type 2 diabetes are further heightened by the fact that it constitutes a risk factor for other

---

35   Theorists note that these distinctions are not that clear-cut: the biophysical, psychological and socio-cultural context of illness/disease are intricately linked. More, crucially, in the Akan language – the dominant language I have used in most of my research – there is no distinction between illness and disease. The Akan term 'yare' applies to a holistic integration of disease and illness.

36   WHO Diabetes Factsheet (Available at http://www.who.int/mediacentre/factsheets/fs312/en/); See also Appendix 3

37   Hereafter, all references to diabetes will refer to type 2 diabetes.

serious chronic diseases such as stroke and heart disease. It is also associated with tuberculosis and HIV/AIDS treatment.

Ghanaians with type 2 diabetes define the condition as a disease with variations in technical understanding of the outlined medical terms, depending on educational level.

> "What I have heard the doctor say is that everyone has something in their stomach and when there is a blockage, it brings about diabetes"

> "The end result is that your body is not producing enough insulin or not utilizing it. There are two forms they say: one that comes on before the age of 40 between ages 1–40 and the type 2 is the one that comes after 40."

But they also define the condition as an illness, drawing largely on social logic.

In a study of acute illness beliefs in a Cameroonian village, the anthropologist Gery Wayne Ryan (1998) observed that for this community:

> "illnesses are alive and animated. They grow, they move, they eat (chop) and have likes and dislikes. People do not have illness; rather illness catches, holds or comes to them".

The majority of Ghanaians with diabetes we have studied, speak of diabetes in a similar way, as an alive, animated and highly demanding visitor:

> "diabetes does not like hunger, it does not like fullness";
> "diabetes does not like music";
> "diabetes does not care about these things"
> "diabetes is a destroyer of the body".

An older woman in a focus group in Kintampo in 2010 made this statement, sarcastically, to loud laughter in the group:

> "what kind of disease is this? You wake up one day and your body is burning. You wake up the next and your mouth is twisted. Diabetes is a bad disease"

The physical and psychological self - what anthropologists like Helman (2000) and Scheper-Hughes and Locke (1987) refer to as the 'body-self'[38] - is the home for this visitor. The visitor brings a daily barrage of physical problems that affects major body areas: eyes, fingers, feet, legs, back, stomach, skin, breasts (for women) and genitals (for women and men). The visitor also wreaks emotional havoc, with fear, unhappiness and anger constituting the major feelings most people experience on a daily basis. Throughout one's life experience with diabetes, these physical and emotional demands occur, in varying levels of intensity. For those who live with diabetes and one or more conditions, the physical and emotional disruptions are even more complex and intense. Essentially, they have to deal with multiple animated visitors with the attendant problems of which visitor to privilege and how. As one elderly woman with diabetes, hypertension, and post-stroke complications, said of her everyday life:

> I always think of why one person like me should contract three different kinds of illnesses. I can't also see properly and can't walk so it really bothers me a lot... but the fact that one person like myself has three different types of diseases... It really bothers me.

Beyond the physical and emotional, diabetes also makes spiritual, social and financial demands (see Figure 7).

---

38   This anthropological notion of the body-self , the relationship between the physical and psychological body (Helman, 2000) lies at the heart of lay conceptions of the body in health and illness. Similar definitions of the intricate relationship between "the objective biological body and the lived body, the body as it is subjectively experienced" are proposed in the literature on the phenomenology of chronic illness (Carel, 2007, p.96)

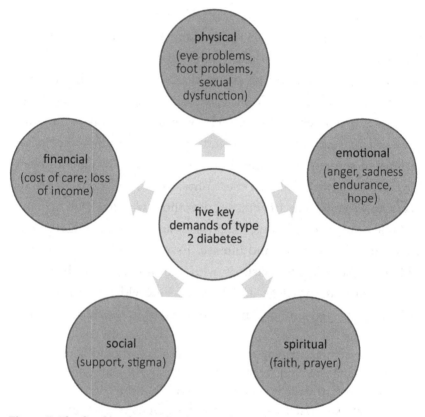

Figure 7. The five key demands of type 2 diabetes

Generally, we can categorise long term Ghanaian diabetes experience in three stages.

Stage 1 is the first encounter with diabetes, when one is diagnosed. Here, everyone is hit emotionally by the diagnosis and everybody struggles psychologically, whether in Accra, Kumasi, Kintampo, London or Berlin, whether wealthy or poor, young or old. Individuals may be in denial, they will seek multiple opinion and advice; they will doctor shop and healershop. This psychological struggle (and corresponding health seeking behaviour) is universal, according to the African and global literature on diabetes experiences[39].

---

39   Campbell et al, 2003.

Stage 2 is the period of adjustment, a period of a year or a year and a half, where one begins to understand the condition, one's body and how to manage the physical, emotional and other demands. Fundamentally diabetes is a physical illness and must be managed typically through medication, diet and exercise. The financial demands of diabetes arise through the cost of care. Most individuals struggle with the financial burden of costs of medicines, diagnostic tests and recommended diets.

I buy medicines for my mother and we spend GHC420 (approximately $107[40]) a month on five essential medicines – Glucophage, Amaryl, Crestor, Exforge HCT, Cardio-aspirin (I use the brand names). None of these medicines are on the list of the National Health Insurance Scheme (NHIS). During the months where medical check-ups are needed, with the full range of diagnostic tests, we spend just over GHC1000 ($255) a month. When my father was with us, we spent at least twice this amount per month. And during the last few months of my father's life we spent an additional GHC3000 ($766) per month on 24-hour nursing care, nursing supplies and physiotherapy. These amounts are what health economists call catastrophic out-of-pocket health expenditure: and this is a common story in many Ghanaian and African households affected by NCDs. It has been estimated that 60% of healthcare is financed out of pocket in low and middle-income countries, compared with 20% in high-income countries[41].

At another level people struggle with diet management: what to eat, how much to eat, when to eat. There are no standard guidelines for diabetes diet management in Ghana and especially for our staple starchy foods. So people ask: do I eat a ball of kenkey or half? How many fingers of plantain should I eat? How thin should my slices of yam be?

40   Based on 2016 US Dollar (USD$) – Ghana Cedi (GHC) exchange rates

41   de-Graft Aikins and Agyemang, 2017.

As individuals attempt to make sense of the condition, healer-shopping can intensify, especially when education, understanding and care are poor. But this is also a period where one can come to terms with one's condition. Across the world, most people with diabetes 'body-listen' that is, they become attuned to the way their body feels in line with rising or diminishing levels of blood-sugar[42]. This emphatic statement was made by a middle aged wealthy man in Accra in an interview:

> "I know my body more than any doctor, so when I feel that it [the diabetes] is going bad then I increase the dosage or lower it"

His statement is one that is reported in the global diabetes literature. However there is a crucial difference between body listening in Ghana and in high income countries of Europe and North America. Many Ghanaians do not have the back-up of actual objective testing, through the diabetes tester kit. So body-listening can lead one down a path of complications because of the near identical nature of 'hypoglycaemic' and 'hyperglycaemic' symptoms (see Figure 8).

symtoms of hyperglycaemia	symptoms of hypoglycaemia
• Being very thirsty • Urinating often • *Feeling very hungry* • Losing weight • *Being very tired* • Dry itchy skin • Slow healing sores • Tingling in the feet • Losing feeling in the feet • Blurry eyesight	• Feeling weak • Feeling confused • Feeling irritable • *Feeling hungry* • *Feeling tired* • Being sweaty • Having a headaches • Passing out • Having a seizure

Figure 8. Symptoms of hyperglycaemia and hypoglycaemia

---

42   Body-listening or body monitoring involves 'knowing the body's unique responses and accurately predicting and interpreting these responses' (Paterson, Thorne, and Dewis 1998). Body-listening is reported in a number of social contexts within and outside Africa (Campbell et al. 2003; Hjelm and Mufunda, 2010).

Stage 3 is the stage of living well or living a transformed life with diabetes. We see this among people who have lived with diabetes for 5 years and over. They have come to terms with the condition, they are more medically adherent and less inclined to healershop, largely because they have experienced the negative effects. However, even within this group, the hope for a cure never fades. As two elderly men I interviewed for my doctoral thesis observed:

"I'm an unhappy host, but it [diabetes] is here and I have to live with it."

"ah well, what I said from the beginning – if you can tell us there is a medicine that will cure you today today we'll all draw to it. Otherwise, we'll go by it [managing diabetes], you see. I know that is what is taking me to my grave"

What are the implications for long-term experience?

Generally, what one should work towards is a healthy quality life with diabetes. *This is possible.* Medical sociologists and social psychologists have given us the most useful concepts to understand long-term experience with chronic disease. They teach us that after the initial disruption of diagnosis and early years of struggle, an individual can experience biographical flow or biographical transformation[43]. Biographical flow occurs when chronic illness slots into the normal flow of life of the sufferer. Biographical transformation occurs when chronic illness leads to a transformation of life in a positive way.

In my research I have tried to identify what enables Ghanaians with diabetes reach these ideal points. Most Ghanaians with diabetes live in a state of biographical flow. As one research participant observed: *"Sickness comes and goes so you can say you are normal."* Few individuals transition into biographical transformation. Those who do, speak of spiritual transformation, in the sense that diabetes

---

43   Carel, 2007; Charmaz, 1983; Reeve et al, 2010.

leads them to a deeper engagement in Christian faith. Individuals either change church affiliation, moving from orthodox churches to charismatic churches or begin an active journey of daily prayer and shunning prior material and social concerns (see Opanin's story in Appendix 5).

The lessons here are these. Given the rising number of people with diabetes, the struggles with treatment and management, the risk of complications and premature death, the challenge is how we help people live good quality long lives with diabetes and co-morbid conditions. But to maintain biographical flow, one needs money to be able to manage the condition effectively[44]. One needs social support. And finally, one needs the appropriate psychological attitude, because without attitudes like acceptance and commitment to medical adherence, no amount of money and unconditional love will be effective.

We need to draw from successful lives with chronic illness: those who have achieved biographical flow and biographical transformation. They are the ones, who in other countries, become 'expert patients' or run 'self-help groups' and transform the landscape of chronic experience and care for themselves and for others[45]. We will see what exists in Ghana and how this can be harnessed for improved experience and care.

---

44   The disability and premature deaths that occur usually do so under conditions of poverty. But as co-morbidities occur and complications persist, the cost of care increases for everyone. And while we have a financial protection scheme with the NHIS, this does not cover all the medical needs of people with chronic conditions.

45   An Expert Patient is "a person who has been empowered with the skills, confidence and knowledge needed to play an active role in making informed decisions about their own health care and management of their chronic condition" (Lightfoot, 2003). One of the earliest definitions of self-help groups was offered by Katz (1981): "Self-help groups are voluntary small group structures for mutual aid and the accomplishment of a special purpose. They are usually formed by peers who have come together for mutual assistance in satisfying a common need, overcoming a common handicap of life-disrupting problem, and bringing about desired social and/or personal change. The initiators and members of such groups perceive that

The Psychology of Chronic Disease Care

The social psychologist Alan Radley makes the important point, that people with chronic illness "live with illness in a world of health"[46]. Individuals do not only respond to the physical event of illness, but they also draw on shared ideas circulating within society about the body, health, illness, life and death. The demands of chronic illness are not matters solely for sufferers – they also become focal points for social perceptions, responses and relationships – some good (like social support), some bad (like stigma). The changes a chronically ill individual goes through can have a profound impact on shared experiences, role expectations and identities within the individual's family, workplace and communities of significance[47]. Within the world of health is the world of care and the world of care has two important groups: caregivers and healthcare providers.

The world of caregivers

The anthropologist John M. Janzen, coined the term 'therapy managing group' to describe the family support system of sick individuals[48]. The therapy managing group made decisions at every stage of the disease course, even though they had no specialized knowledge of disease or therapy. Families continue to play a significant role in the care of sick individuals in many African countries and particularly so when sicknesses are chronic or terminal. For most Ghanaians with diabetes, we have studied, there is at least one person in the family who provides care beyond the ordinary:

---

their needs are not, or cannot be, met by or through existing social institutions"

46   Radley, 1994, p. 136.

47   As Crossley (2000:82) notes: "shattered assumptions regarding the future and one's body means that the person living with illness feels profoundly alienated from the world of other people".

48   Janzen, 1982

this person will buy the medicines, manage and supervise healthcare visits, cook, clean, bathe and carry, depending on the seriousness of the condition. This person does so out of love (e.g a spouse, a child, a sibling) or out of duty because they are nominated to do so by the broader family. For those with serious complications or co-morbidities or for the very elderly, having a primary care giver is crucial. But caregivers need care and support too, we are discovering. They also live with the demands of diabetes I described earlier – the aches and pains of lifting and carrying, the emotional tensions and turmoil that come with watching a loved one shun treatment or deteriorate, the financial stresses of everyday and emergency treatment and so on. Often the disruptions experienced by both sufferer and caregiver can lead to tensions and damage relationships. As illness progresses and cost of care increases some families can abandon their chronically ill relatives. For some people with diabetes, family members are therefore not 'therapy managers'. Instead they are 'therapy damagers', people with bad minds who cause illness and illness complications (through sorcery and witchcraft) and other negative outcomes (through social undermining and abandonment).

Family support and caregiving is crucial, but it can be double-edged and needs careful management across the life course. The lives and psychological needs of caregivers need to be better understood to inform the development of appropriate interventions for both the chronically ill and caregivers[49]. We need, in particular, to do more research on the damaging effects of supernatural attributions on family life.

---

49   The two family case studies presented in Appendix 6 and Appendix 7 describe opposite extremes of diabetes caregiving in Ghana: the ideal, which several families struggle with; and the difficult, which mirrors the experience of many poor families.

The world of healthcare providers

The second group in the 'world of care' is healthcare providers. And in Ghana we have a vibrant pluralistic healthcare system made up of biomedicine (our regular doctors, nurses, pharmacists, laboratory technicians, care workers), ethnomedicine (herbalists, faith healers, shrine priests [or fetish priests]) and the Complementary and Alternative Medicine sector (or CAM for short, made up of Chinese medicine, Indian medicine, chiropractors, etc). Sixteen years ago, when I first interviewed healthcare providers for my PhD, the same categories existed although there were fewer numbers per category. However their ideologies haven't changed. Biomedicine says we manage disease, ethnomedicine says we cure disease, and CAM oscillates between management and cure depending on condition.

A senior medical doctor said this to me in an interview in 2001:
"The traditional healers do not advertise treatment for hypercholesterolaemia (high cholesterol in the blood). Yeah, they don't advertise treatment for hypercholesterolaemia for the simple reason that they don't hear a lot spoken about it. But let me get up today and get on the air and let me sort of set up an association for lipid disorders and so on and so forth and the traditional healers will find a remedy for it and say that it is curable."

At the time of this interview, Top Herbal had monopoly in media advertising and although shrine priests provided a service they did so in secret. Now there are multiple herbal clinic adverts on radio, TV and in newspapers every day. Drive along the Accra-Kumasi road and there are at least 10 billboards of traditional shrine priests advertising services for a wide range of physical, social and spiritual conditions. I know of famous shrine priests who have websites and some who are flown, business class, to Europe and North America to tend to the medical and social needs of Ghanaian migrants. And most members of the ethnomedical system promise cures, with bolder claims made by the year. One, which appears in the newspapers regularly, claims, in capital letters:

"RECOVER FROM DEMENTIA, STROKE, KIDNEY FAILURE AND PARKINSON IN JUST 3 WEEKS OR 100% OF YOUR MONEY BACK. STRICTLY WITHOUT SURGERY."

And what does the miracle treatment involve?

"World's No 1 massage!"

Well, these claims are simply not true. I focus on the issue of cure because cure is a recurrent hope in the lives of many people with diabetes and other chronic diseases[50]. This makes the cure industry of herbalists and faith healers, powerful and legitimate in their psychological life. And we must understand that psychological need and deal with it. But we must also understand that when hope for a cure meets claims to cure in the herbal and faith healing sectors the outcome can be catastrophic with complications and premature death being common.

Healershopping will always occur, within and across sectors, because chronic disease is long term and life and health needs evolve. Medical pluralism will continue to be a central model of healthcare in Ghana for the long term as long as there are complex illnesses that biomedicine cannot cure and as long as our social logic on risk and treatment is cognitive polyphasic.

---

50   See Appendix 8 for Opanin's story

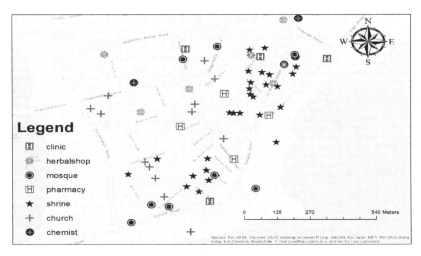

Figure 9. Medical pluralism in Ga Mashie, Accra

Figure 9 shows the spatial distribution of pluralistic health services in Ga Mashie, where I have been engaged in long-term chronic disease research, since 2010. The map shows 61 facilities: 1 polyclinic, 2 private clinics, 6 private pharmacies, 3 chemical shops, 14 churches, 8 mosques and 27 traditional shrines. Of the 61 facilities, only 1 is government owned. Individuals use these centres, but they also seek treatment from outside their community in Osu, Kaneshie, East Legon and services beyond Accra[51].

In my own family, we have used 20 healthcare providers over a ten year period, including specialists, diagnostic services and pharmacies. Some of these providers were situated in East Legon (where my parents live) and others in Airport, Achimota, Labone, Osu and Korle-Bu. And when my mother got to the end of her

---

51   The map of medical pluralism in Ga Mashie is, of course, static. It does not show the dynamic and chaotic (visually and auditorily) elements of mobile health services: the itinerant BP and weight measurers who offer door to door services, the itinerant herbal salesman or woman, or the Agbeve Tonic van that drives slowly through neighbourhoods all day with blaring megaphones.

tether she went as far as a herbalist in Swedru – who claimed to be able to cure hypertension and stroke - causing a major family crisis.

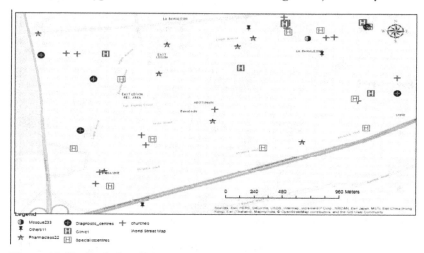

Figure 10. Medical pluralism in East Legon, Accra

Figure 10 shows a concentration of pluralistic services in a small enclave of East Legon (bounded by Shiashie, Okponglo and the A&C Mall road): 12 specialist centres, 5 clinics, 5 diagnostic centres, 9 pharmacies, 12 churches, 1 mosque and 3 health advocacy organizations. Most of these services did not exist when my family journey began in 2005. Some of these services, it is important to note, are private sector services managed by specialists employed in the public sector. Crucially, the two maps highlight disparities between systems of care in poor and wealthy neighbourhoods. There are more traditional healing systems in Ga Mashie compared to biomedical services. In East Legon, there are more biomedical services – and high end specialist services – compared to traditional healing systems.

Ghana's healthcare system is fragmented and the cure industry thrives because of this. What is clearly required is greater understanding of the nuances in the cure industry, in order to regulate effectively. There are certain facts we know. We know that traditional medicine has always been creative. In the colonial era, anthropologists documented the flexibility, ability and power of West and East African healers to 'invent tradition' in order to move with changing times and socio-cultural demands[52]. Their manipulation of the mass media and public spaces these days should therefore not be surprising. Nor should the fact that many are developing hyphenated identities, as herbalist-prophets and herbalist-apostles. Given Ghana's current hyper-religious environment, these creative healers know that layering cure claims with faith claims is more powerful than pharmacological cure in isolation.

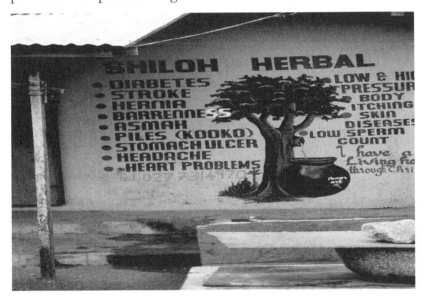

Curing chronic diseases with herbal medicines and "a living hope through Christ"

To summarise, two key insights emerge on the psychology of care. First, care represents the complex intersection of the person with diabetes, the family, community (of significance) and the health system. Care goes beyond the individual, can disrupt the lives of primary caregivers and impoverish families. It shows that not

---

52   See Last, 1992; and Rekdal, 1999.

preventing and not treating our conditions properly have major knock on effects on all of us. The effects are financial, physical, psychological and spiritual. Secondly, the quest for a cure is costly, financially, psychologically and medically.

The solution to the problems of care goes beyond psychology. We must, of course, understand the psyche and motivations of the cure industry – the stuff of psychology – but we must also regulate the industry because we have sufficient evidence of their harmful effects on vulnerable people, and this is the stuff of health, fiscal and legal policies.

PART 3: CURING OUR ILLS?

Understanding Our Physical and Ideological Ills

Can we cure our ills? The answer is mixed. Our physical and ideological ills are intertwined and must be dealt with as such. If we return to our social psychological conceptual framework, we see, firstly, that chronic illness risk, experience and care are nested in the four levels of social organization (see figure 11). Each phenomenon operates at all four levels, but at each level, the phenomenon is different. Risk operates at the four levels, through natural, social, structural, supernatural casual theories. Experience operates at four levels through the physical, emotional, spiritual, social and financial demands of illness. Care highlights the complex relationship between the chronically ill individual, primary caregiver, social attitudes, and pluralistic health systems. An important feature of chronic disease risk, experience and care in Ghana, is the way the spiritual/supernatural operates at all levels of social organization, as a cause and consequence of serious illness. This feature requires more critical inter-disciplinary research.

Secondly, we also see the importance of "conceptualis[ing], simultaneously, both the power of society and the agency of individuals" for improving experience and care.

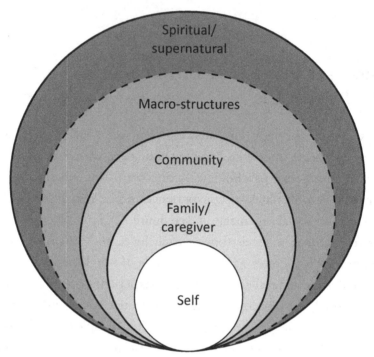

Figure 11. Chronic disease risk, experience and care in multi-level nested relationships

Let us extend our previous exercise on love to diabetes experience (see figure 12). Say Kwame and Akua did get married, after all, and Kwame now has diabetes (because as I'm sure you have gathered Akua is a Fantse woman who specialises in '*nchichiwee*'[53]). So Kwame has diabetes (this is the intrapersonal level). He lives his life in a world of health in which his relationship with his primary caregiver, Akua, matters (this is the interpersonal level). The quality of social support he receives from significant social groups, such as the church members he has grown up with from the youth choir days to men's fellowship, matters (the positional/social level). Finally, the quality and cost of healthcare he receives matter, whether he adheres

---

53   Colloquial Fante term for fried snacks and foods.

strictly to biomedical care or he healershops within the traditional medicine and faith healing sectors (the structural level).

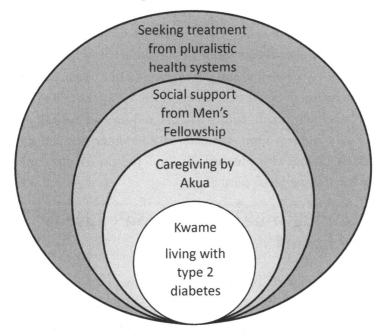

Figure 12. Diabetes care at four levels of analysis

The power of society in this example encompasses the positives and negatives of a world of health. Individual agency would be Kwame's ability to attain biographical flow or biographical transformation, inspite of the power of society, for example negative social attitudes or prohibitive medical treatment.

Our ideological ills are complex but well documented. Ghana's formal biomedical system is under-resourced and overstretched and healthcare is not accessible and equitable for many. Due to a long history of engagement with infectious disease, biomedical systems are ideologically oriented towards privileging time-limited treatment and cure over prevention and long-term illness management. Relations between national health policymakers and powerful actors in global development and health communities are unequal and health policies and interventions are too often driven by external interests rather than by local evidence and needs. As a result minimal investments have been made in the human and material resources required to prevent and control NCDs. Prevalence rates of preventable chronic conditions continue to grow exponentially, as are rates of disability and premature deaths from conditions which are managed better in countries with stronger health systems.

Fundamentally, then, 'curing our ills' requires addressing all the levels, and it requires a transformational encounter between agentic individuals (living with physical ills) and the power structures in society (that shape ideological ills).

Developing multi-level chronic disease interventions

Global health experts make a strong argument for NCD patient advocacy. They draw attention to the fact that the political momentum that transformed HIV/AIDS care globally was driven by the advocacy of people with HIV/AIDS, activists and volunteers. They note that "people living with NCDs need champions to advocate for the cause or be activists themselves" in order to move global and local NCDs policies from rhetoric to action[54].

In 2010, I co-published a comparative review of existing NCD interventions in Ghana and Cameroon, with a Cameroonian colleague, Professor Lem Atanga and British colleague Dr Petra Boynton[55]. What we found in Ghana was an emerging movement of self-help groups for diabetes, cancers, heart disease and mental disorders. Some were established by chronically ill individuals themselves. Most offered education and moral support for members, and some lobbied government and funders for improved care. All of them had

54   Mendis and Chestnov, 2016, p206.
55   de-Graft Aikins, Boynton and Atanga, 2010.

insufficient funds and logistical resources to transform the landscape of NCD care in the long-term. These movements were evolving within a policy context characterised by rhetoric and inaction.

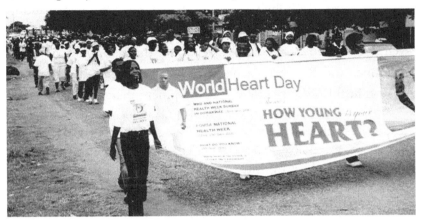

March for World Heart Day

Ghana has an NCD policy that was launched in 2012 after a 15-year consultative process, in which I participated[56]. The policy ticks all the global NCD policy benchmarks. But it remains on paper, with no funding for implementation. My experience with national and international NCD policy development teaches me to expect a protracted delay with policy implementation, as we see for policies on disability and mental health[57].

Given the rhetorical policy climate we have in Ghana, NCD advocacy should be an option we vigorously pursue. We can learn from countries like Cameroon, Mauritius, Rwanda and Brazil, where, despite limited resources, bold NCD policies have been implemented with strong community-based action[58].

---

56   National Policy for the Prevention and Control of Chronic Non-communicable Diseases, 2012

57   Persons with Disability Act715 launched in 2006; Ghana Mental Health Act 846 launched in 2012

58   See Appendix 3 for a synthesis of best practices in NCD prevention and control in LMICs.

CONCLUSIONS

I have two critical psychology mentors: my former PhD supervisor, Professor Cathy Campbell, a South African, and Professor Sandra Jovchelovitch, a Brazilian. Both are based at the Department of Psychological and Behavioural Sciences at the London School of Economics and Political Science. They observed, in a highly cited paper on health, community and development that:

> "in our countries of origin Brazil and South Africa where debates between theory and practice, social theory and social change, psychology and social justice have long taken place.... [there has been] the vital need to link theory and practice without undermining either. [This approach] also stresses how much can be learned from concrete and practical interventions where theories are put into use and...how fertile they are not only in pointing towards ways of understanding the world but also in changing it"[59]

I have spent the best part of 16 years studying chronic illness experiences through a critical psychology lens and understanding the political economy of NCD policy through practical engagement with policy communities. Over the period, I have returned repeatedly to a gut instinct that the best thing to do in Ghana is to empower communities and individuals at risk to prevent illnesses in the first place. Because once illness becomes a reality, individuals are at the mercy of complex local and global forces and for the poor, premature death is all too common[60]. This means for those of us in

---

59 Campbell and Jovchelovitch, 2000, p.268

60 The danger then is a normalization of death and dying in epidemic proportions. The popular Ghanaian slogan *all die be die* is not a mere slogan. It has become a social representation of 'acceptable death' that is creating a new social reality of self-destructive health and social behaviours. The representation blurs the line between longstanding cultural representations about 'good death' and 'bad death' (see van der Geest, 2004). The health and social behaviours raise the risk of illnesses and premature deaths, particularly in poor and marginalised communities.

this Great Hall who are at risk of getting the major NCDs, we need to know our NCD status and we need to eat better, manage our weight, be physically active, reduce alcohol intake and stop smoking, if we are smoking[61]. For those of us who already live with chronic conditions, the rising cost of care and the reality of family tensions and disintegration means we need an NCD-competent NHIS, to absorb the cost of care, and regulated social care interventions for all. At present there is a growing - and unregulated - nursing care industry that caters largely for the wealthy. We need affordable options for the less wealthy. For those of us caring for loved ones with chronic conditions, we need support and family-oriented social care interventions will be beneficial to us.

Over the last 6 years, my independent work has centred on a longitudinal social psychological study of diabetes experiences in Ga Mashie, Accra. Last year I began work with a multidisciplinary group of Legon researchers and students from population studies, psychology and pharmacy, as well as community health nurses, to establish a hypertension control project, called *Tsui Anaa* (Take Heart), in Ga Mashie. Both projects will evolve into the establishment of self-help groups for hypertension and diabetes run jointly by community members the UG team and community health workers. We are using a blend of patient advocacy and community conscientization approaches and plan to study the progress of the groups over the next few years, cost the process and extend the model to other communities. What I am working towards is building an interdisciplinary project - rooted in theory and practice - that will enhance my understanding of community health, train students and healthcare workers and benefit Ghanaian communities in need.

---

61   See Appendix 3 for notes on WHO endorsed NCD prevention strategies.

ACKNOWLEDGEMENTS

Mr Chair, I would like to conclude with brief acknowledgements. I did not arrive at this stage of my scholarly journey alone. I have a host of important people to thank. My mentors who gave me a strong foundation and compass: some of whom I have mentioned during my lecture, but others at Legon I need to mention by name – Professor Francis Dodoo, Professor Kweku Osam, Professor C. Charles Mate-Kole, Professor Kwadwo Koram and Professor Mary Esther Dakubu. My research collaborators and colleagues with whom I have built a body of research; My graduate students who drive my passion to teach and mentor and my new group of postdoctoral mentees with whom I can chart new scholarly adventures (and I must acknowledge Dr Adriana Biney, Dr Ernestina Dankyi and Dr Antoinette Tsiboe-Darko for their support as I prepared for this lecture).

The Regional Institute for Population Studies is my academic home. But I have had the honour of serving the Centre for Social Policy Studies, as director and the School of Graduate Studies, as Vice Dean. I would like to thank my RIPS, CSPS and SGS colleagues for their support.

I am deeply thankful for my family and friends who have provided support and sanctuary for decades; and to my husband, Yaw Awuku Boohene, who has been my keenest lay critic, always pushing me to answer the 'so what' question. I would like to acknowledge the presence of my old Wesley Girls' High School headmistress, Dr (Mrs) Rosina Acheampong, an inspirational woman whose life of service embodies our school motto: Live Pure, Speak True, Right Wrongs and Follow the King.

I would also like to emphasise my gratitude to you, Mr Chairman, for supporting the career development of early career scholars at Legon. I am a beneficiary of this visionary and vital investment. And I feel privileged to have been given the opportunity of this inaugural platform under your chairmanship.

I dedicate my lecture to my beloved parents: my father Mr Seth Kwamina Baisie de-Graft Aikins, who should have been here this evening, and my mother Mrs Eleanor Nana Sar de-Graft Aikins, who is right here.

Thank you all for your kind attention.

APPENDICES

Appendix 1: Research projects and locations in Ghana, 1997 – 2016.

1a. Map of Ghana showing research areas

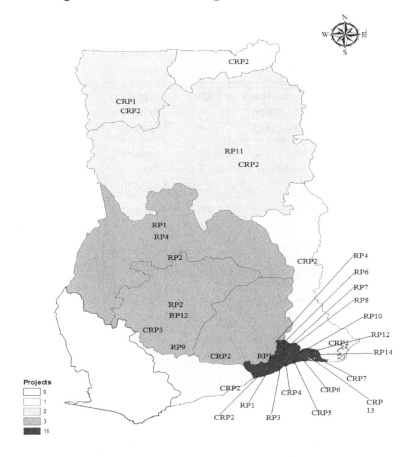

1b. Funded Research projects on core research areas.

Project identifier	Project	Year/du-ration	Region(s)	Location
Research Project 1 (RP1)	Social representations of diabetes (PhD research)	2000-2001	Greater Accra Region Brong Ahafo Region Eastern Region	Accra, Tema Kintampo, Nkoranza Aburi
RP2	Postdoc pilot study on toxic nutrition *(funded by ESRC)*	2005	Brong Ahafo Region	Nkoranza
RP3	Food beliefs and practices during pregnancy	2006-2007	Greater Accra Region	Accra
RP4	Art and mental health project	2009-2010	Greater Accra Region	Pantang Hospital
RP5	Social Representations of diabetes (PhD research follow up)	2010	Brong Ahafo Region	Kintampo
RP6	Social representations of diabetes in an urban poor community	2010 – present	Greater Accra Region	Ga Mashie
RP7	NYU-RIPS Task shifting project (funded by NYU)	2011-2012	Greater Accra Region	Ga Mashie
RP8	NYU-RIPS twin cities project (funded by NYU)	2011-2012	Greater Accra Region	Ga Mashie

Project identifier	Project	Year/duration	Region(s)	Location
RP9	RODAM (funded by the European Commission)	2011 - 2014	Ashanti Region [London, Amsterdam, Berlin]	Kumasi, Obuasi (and surrounding rural communities)
RP10	Social protection project (funded by PASGR)	2013-2014	Greater Accra Region	Accra; Ga Mashie
RP11	Scaling up mental health services project (funded by GCC)	2014-2015	Northern Region	Mamprugu Moaduri, North Gonja and West Mamprusi Districts
RP12	CID Project (funded by Duke University)	2015-2016	Greater Accra Region Ashanti Region	Accra Kumasi
RP13	HTN intervention project (funded by ORID, UG)	2015-2016	Greater Accra Region	Ga Mashie
RP14	Mental Health and Development (funded by NYU-GIPH)	2016-present	Greater Accra Region	Selected schools in Accra

1c. Field-based commissioned research

Project identifier	Project	Year/du-ration	Region	Location
Commis-sioned Research Project 1 (CRP1)	Alcohol use and epilepsy *(commis-sioned by DANIDA)*	1997	Upper West	Wa (and selected communities)
CRP2	RHN review *(commis-sioned by the Ministry of Health, MOH)*	2007	Greater Accra Eastern Volta Central Northern Upper East Upper West	Amasaman, Akim-Oda Hohoe, Keta Asikuma-Odo-beng-Brakwa Tamale, Gushegu Bolgatanga Wa
CRP3	MVP Project *(Commis-sioned by Overseas De-velopment Institute, ODI)*	2008	Ashanti	Amansie West District
CRP4	IOB project *(Commis-sioned by IOB)*	2009-2010	Greater Accra Eastern	Accra Atiwa, Birim North, and Kwahu South Districts

Project identifier	Project	Year/duration	Region	Location
CRP5	Alliance project *(Commissioned by World Health Organisation, WHO)*	2009-2010	Greater Accra	Accra
CRP6	WHO/LSE HPSR Study *(Commissioned by WHO)*	2009-2010	Greater Accra	Accra
CRP7	FAO project *(Commissioned by Food and Agricultural Organization, FAO)*	2014-2015	Greater Accra	Accra

Appendix 2. Cognitive polyphasia: employing diverse and opposite ways of thinking

Social Representations Theory was developed through Serge Moscovici's pioneering study of social representations of psychoanalysis in 1950s France. In this study Moscovici described how French social groups of different ages, classes and professions anchored the new idea of 'psychoanalysis' - introduced by Sigmund Freud - into existing systems of knowledge about medicine and therapy[62]. Moscovici observed that, in constructing representations of psychoanalysis, the relationship and relevance of psychoanalysis to the practical lives of individuals, shaped their structures and processes of thinking about the phenomenon. Thus, religion, science, political ideology and common sense were drawn on eclectically, interchangeably and often in contradictory ways, across social groups and within individual minds. Moscovici referred to this thinking process as cognitive polyphasia. He defined it as the "dynamic co-existence – interference or specialisation - of the distinct modalities of knowledge, corresponding to definite relations between man and his environment"[63]. He deemed this "tendency to employ diverse and even opposite ways of thinking...[as] a normal state of affairs in ordinary life and communication"[64].

This observation - that everyday knowledge is necessarily complex and sometimes conflicting, that we may draw on these with relative ease in some moments or with tension in others - is well documented in the anthropological literature. This phenomenon has been described in terms of the way some African communities incorporate traditional medicine and biomedical ideologies into cultural healing repertoires and on how Cameroonians with diabetes or Tanzanians with hypertension make sense of their conditions[65]. It points to the everyday use of available systems of social knowledge for meaningful and functional purposes. My interest lies in the way these complex, yet fluid, thinking-feeling processes inform individuals understanding of diabetes and other chronic conditions, and ensuing health behaviours and illness actions[66]

---

62   Moscovici, 2008.

63   Moscovici, 2008, p.190.

64   Moscovici, 2008, p.245

65   See Feierman and Janzen, 1992; Goody, 1975; Rekdal, 1999; Awah et al, 2008a, 2008b; Strahl, 2003.

66   See de-Graft Aikins, 2012

Appendix 3. WHO endorsed strategies to reduce risks of NCDs

WHO states: "Common, preventable risk factors underlie most non-communicable diseases. Most non-communicable diseases are the result of four particular behaviours (tobacco use, physical inactivity, unhealthy diet, and the harmful use of alcohol) that lead to four key metabolic/physiological changes (raised blood pressure, overweight/obesity, raised blood glucose and raised cholesterol)." (WHO, http://www.who.int/gho/ncd/risk_factors/en/)

Common, preventable (modifiable) risk factors	Metabolic/physiological changes
Harmful use of alcohol [67]:	Raised cholesterol [68]
"Harmful use of alcohol is a pattern of drinking that is already causing damage to health. The damage may be either physical (e.g., liver damage from chronic drinking) or mental (e.g., depressive episodes secondary to drinking).	High total serum cholesterol, defined as ≥ 6.2 millimoles per litre (mmol/l) (240 milligrams per decilitre, mg/dl), for adults from 40 to 79 years of age.
Hazardous use of alcohol is a pattern of alcohol consumption that carries a risk of harmful consequences to the drinker. These include damage to physical or mental health and/or social consequences to the drinker or others."	Raised cholesterol increases the risks of heart disease and stroke.

67   Babor and Higgins-Biddle, 2001.
68   WHO, Raised cholesterol. Available at http://www.who.int/gho/ncd/risk_factors/cholesterol_text/en/

Common, preventable (modifiable) risk factors	Metabolic/physiological changes
Low-risk use of alcohol: - No more than two standard drinks* a day - Do *not* drink at least two days of the week *A standard drink is: - 1 can of ordinary beer (330ml at 5%) - 1 single shot of spirits (whisky, gin, vodka, etc) (40ml at 40%) - 1 glass of wine or a small glass of sherry (140ml at 12%) - 1 small glass of liquer or aperitif (70ml at 25%) *Note that there are times when even one or two drinks can be too much:* - When driving or operating machinery. - When pregnant or breast feeding. - When taking certain medications - If you have certain medical conditions. - If you cannot control your drinking	

Common, preventable (modifiable) risk factors	Metabolic/physiological changes
Unhealthy diet[8]: Consuming more foods high in energy, fats, free sugars or salt/sodium, and not eating enough fruit, vegetables and dietary fibre such as whole grains. A healthy diet consists of[9]: • "Fruits, vegetables, legumes (e.g. lentils, beans), nuts and whole grains (e.g. unprocessed maize, millet, oats, wheat, brown rice). • At least 400 g (5 portions) of fruits and vegetables a day (2). Potatoes, sweet potatoes, cassava and other starchy roots are not classified as fruits or vegetables. • Less than 50 g (or around 12 level teaspoons) of free sugars for a person of healthy body weight. (Note: Most free sugars are added to foods or drinks by the manufacturer, cook or consumer, and can also be found in sugars naturally present in honey, syrups, fruit juices and fruit juice concentrates)	Raised blood glucose or hyperglycaemia[10] Hyperglycaemia, or raised blood sugar, is a common effect of uncontrolled diabetes. For adults aged 18 and above, raised blood glucose is defined as fasting plasma glucose concentration of 7.0 mmol/l (126 mg/dl) or being on medication for raised blood glucose. Over time raised blood glucose/diabetes leads to serious damage to many of the body's systems, including the heart, blood vessels, eyes, kidneys, and nerves. • Adults with diabetes have a two- to three-fold increased risk of heart attacks and strokes • Combined with reduced blood flow, neuropathy (nerve damage) in the feet increases the chance of foot ulcers, infection and eventual need for limb amputation.

69   WHO Fact sheet N°394 on Healthy Diet (Updated September 2015) http://www.who.int/mediacentre/factsheets/fs394/en/
70   WHO Fact sheet N°394 on Healthy Diet (Updated September 2015) http://www.who.int/mediacentre/factsheets/fs394/en/
71   WHO Diabetes mellitus Fact sheet N°138 (Available at http://www.who.int/mediacentre/factsheets/fs138/en/).

Common, preventable (modifiable) risk factors	Metabolic/physiological changes
• Less than 30% of total energy intake from fats. Unsaturated fats (e.g. found in fish, avocado, nuts, sunflower, canola and olive oils) are preferable to saturated fats (e.g. found in fatty meat, butter, palm and coconut oil, cream, cheese, ghee and lard). Industrial trans fats (found in processed food, fast food, snack food, fried food, frozen pizza, pies, cookies, margarines and spreads) are not part of a healthy diet. • Less than 5 g of salt (equivalent to approximately 1 teaspoon) per day and use iodized salt."	• Diabetic retinopathy is an important cause of blindness, and occurs as a result of long-term accumulated damage to the small blood vessels in the retina. • Diabetes is among the leading causes of kidney failure

Common, preventable (modifiable) risk factors	Metabolic/physiological changes
Physical inactivity[72]	Raised blood pressure or Hypertension[73]
"physical activity is any bodily movement produced by skeletal muscles that requires energy expenditure. This includes activities undertaken while working, playing, carrying out household chores, travelling, and engaging in recreational pursuits. PA is not to be confused with 'exercise' which is a subcategory of physical activity that is planned, structured, repetitive, and aims to improve or maintain one or more components of physical fitness". Physical inactivity is a lack of the above.	Raised blood pressure or high blood pressure or hypertension is a condition in which the blood vessels have persistently raised pressure. Blood is carried from the heart to all parts of the body in blood vessels, or arteries. Each time the heart beats, it pumps blood into the vessels. Blood pressure is created by the force of blood pushing against the walls of blood vessels (arteries) as it is pumped by the heart. The higher the pressure the harder the heart has to pump.
To enhance health through physical activity, adults aged 15 – 64, should do the following:	• Normal adult blood pressure: blood pressure of 120 mm Hg* when the heart beats (systolic) and a blood pressure of 80 mm Hg when the heart relaxes (diastolic).
• at least 150 minutes of moderate-intensity physical activity (e.g walking, cycling, doing sports) throughout the week, or do at least 75 minutes of vigorous-intensity physical activity throughout the week, or an equivalent combination of moderate- and vigorous-intensity activity.	• High blood pressure: blood pressure equal to or above 140 mm Hg when the heart beats (systolic) and pressure equal to or above 90 mm Hg when the heart relaxes (diastolic)

72   WHO Physical Activity Factsheet (updated February 2017). Available at http://www.who.int/mediacentre/factsheets/fs385/en/
73   WHO Hypertension. Available at http://www.who.int/topics/hypertension/en/

Common, preventable (modifiable) risk factors	Metabolic/physiological changes
• for additional health benefits, increase their moderate-intensity physical activity to 300 minutes per week, or equivalent. • Muscle-strengthening activities should be done involving major muscle groups on 2 or more days a week. • In order to be beneficial for cardiorespiratory health, all activity should be performed in bouts of at least 10 minutes duration.	The higher the blood pressure, the higher the risk of damage to the heart and blood vessels in major organs such as the brain and kidneys. Hypertension is the most important preventable cause of heart disease and stroke worldwide. Hypertension is known as the "silent killer" because most people with hypertension have no symptoms at all. Sometimes hypertension causes symptoms such as headache, shortness of breath, dizziness, chest pain, palpitations of the heart and nose bleeds. (*blood pressure is measured in millimetres of mercury, mmHg)

Tobacco use[74]	Overweight and obesity[76]
The use of tobacco products such as cigarettes, light cigarettes, menthol cigarettes, cigars and pipes, bidis, kreteks (clove cigarettes), and hookahs (water pipes)[75].	Abnormal or excessive fat accumulation that may impair health.
Tobacco products are products made entirely or partly of leaf tobacco as raw material, which are intended to be smoked, sucked, chewed or snuffed. All tobacco products contain the highly addictive psychoactive ingredient, nicotine.	Body mass index (BMI) is used to classify overweight and obesity in adults. It is defined as a person's weight in kilograms divided by the square of his height in meters (kg/m2). For adults:
Second-hand smoke	• overweight is a BMI greater than or equal to 25; and
'Second-hand smoke is the smoke that fills enclosed public spaces such as offices, restaurants, and nightclubs when people burn tobacco products such as cigarettes, *bidis* and water-pipes. There are more than 4000 chemicals in tobacco smoke. At least 250 are known to be harmful and more than 50 are known to cause cancer.'	• obesity is a BMI greater than or equal to 30. Raised BMI is a major risk factor for the followng NCDs: • cardiovascular diseases (mainly heart disease and stroke) • diabetes;

74 WHO Tobacco factsheet. . Available at http://www.who.int/mediacentre/factsheets/fs339/en/

75 US Department of Health and Human Services, BeTobaccofree.gov. Available at https://betobaccofree.hhs.gov/about-tobacco/ Smoked-Tobacco-Products/index.html

76 WHO Obesity/Overweight Factsheet (updated October, 2017). Available at accessed http://www.who.int/mediacentre/factsheets/fs311/en/)

Tobacco use[74]	Overweight and obesity[76]
"There is no safe level of exposure to second-hand tobacco smoke. In adults, second-hand smoke causes serious cardiovascular and respiratory diseases, including coronary heart disease and lung cancer. In infants, it causes sudden death. In pregnant women, it causes low birth weight."	• musculoskeletal disorders (especially osteoarthritis – a highly disabling degenerative disease of the joints); • some cancers (including endometrial, breast, ovarian, prostate, liver, gallbladder, kidney, and colon).

Appendix 4. Social representations of diabetes: examples from Nkoranza

Two middle-aged sisters in Nkoranza, Maame and Akosua, had diabetes. They also had other sisters who had diabetes. Both Maame and Akosua attributed their diabetes to heredity. As Akosua observed: *"Diabetes runs through my family. Three of my sisters have diabetes. Most of the women on my mother's side of the family have diabetes"*. At the same time they also speculated that their diabetes was at root caused by sorcery.

Maame: *"The disease is not a family disease. It was ((planted)) in the family by witches. According to some sources my mother feasted on somebody's child; after four days the child died. So they used disease to disgrace us. It is not a family disease.*

Here, a distinction was made between a heritable disease that occurred through genetic transfer (via the bloodline) and a disease that affected a family through supernatural means. Their mother had committed an alleged social transgression, witchcraft, the punishment for which had been a chronic disease, which had then been passed down the matrilineal line to affect a group of sisters. This explanation was similar to explanations given for spiritual slaves, such as the girls and women of traditional shrines in the Brong Ahafo, Ashanti, Northern and Volta Regions, who pay for the social transgressions of their fathers or mothers by serving the shrines for the rest of their lives. While these spiritual slaves lost their freedom through shrine servitude, Maame, Akosua and sisters lost theirs through a debilitating chronic disease.

These blended theories did not only reside in the minds of lay individuals. They also resided in the minds of health professionals. When biomedical professionals, in particular, subscribed to supernatural causal theories, this reinforced the social and functional legitimacy of the theories. Afia, a young woman in Nkoranza recounted her experience of diagnosis:

"I didn't know it was that disease so I went [...] and the doctor examined me and saw nothing. One nurse told me that my sickness must be abonsam yare (Satanic illness) and that I should go home and find another means of cure. I became so frightened."

[Source: de-Graft Aikins, 2005b]

Appendix 5. Biographical transformation: Opanin's story

Opanin lived with diabetes and had just recovered from prostate cancer prior to our first interview. Opanin asserted that diabetes had led him to develop a deeper spiritual life. But this faith had come about when diabetic symptoms led to the discovery of prostate cancer, and through the subsequent search for the meaning of his life, when he believed the prostate cancer would kill him.

"Well, one of the symptoms I have is increased water passage, you go to the toilet. And fortunately or rather unfortunately, it was this frequency of water passage that led me to discover that I really had prostrate cancer. [...] I was grateful to diabetes because it [the prostate cancer] was fairly advanced. I had a PSA level of 17 to almost 18 and when you get to 20, it could be very serious". [...] When they diagnosed, it was proved that there was a malignancy. The doctor who read this to me was a very young inexperienced doctor who he went by the book: "17.418 - this is a very aggressive kind of cancer and it's the American Blacks who have it frequently. Why don't you go to America and see what they can do about it for you?" He then went on and on until I asked him, 'So how long do I have?' he said, "oh, the probabilities are for five years." So I said oh, so I don't have more than five years, and I became....if I'm going to die in five years, what should I be doing? Do I begin to write my memoirs or ignore it? So I surveyed my life and didn't think that it was interesting enough to want to write anything about it so at some point in time, I simply gave up.

AdGA: 'Gave up?' What do you mean 'gave up'?

Gave up in the sense that I'm going to die and so I want to go quietly. I don't want to make any waves at all. And I felt the five years were long enough to fade out of the system so that by the time you're dead, nobody remembers you. So I think it was a stupid decision I made, but I made it. I stopped writing. I'd gone to London with the intent to finish a book I had started and I stopped it. I was like please

> if I have to go, I want to go quietly, I don't want to create any offense, I don't want to.... I just wait and see. It was a stupid decision but I made it and then it was a really miraculous intervention. It was when I actually saw a cancer specialist in London. He... after talking to me a while then told me that 'well, do not forget the spiritual side'. So we really went through a spiritual exercise and now I feel strong. It changed my life in a way and now I'm a little more of a Christian than before."

[Source: de-Graft Aikins, 2005b]

Appendix 6. Diabetes and the world of caregiving: John's story

John had lived with diabetes for 15 years and had a longer history of hypertension. John and his family attributed his diabetes to a mix of dietary imbalance, poor lifestyle practices (smoking and drinking), and heredity. Three weeks before the ethnography, he had had a leg amputated. He could not return to his casual post-retirement job as a security guard as a result, and his loss of income had a considerable impact on his family's finances. The family's struggle with a diminished budget was compounded by the ongoing need for expensive insulin treatment and dietary management.

His family was committed to his care, despite the financial constraints. His wife Diane provided round the clock care, and his older daughter Hannah and son Charles took extended time off work to provide secondary care. A daughter who lived abroad sent regular donations to supplement her parents' pension. A young priest and family friend, Patrick, came by regularly to offer John and his family spiritual and moral support. For much of the duration of the fieldwork, John oscillated between depression and anger at his disability, and he often withdrew from making decisions about his medical care and self care. Diane and Hannah, therefore, took active daily control of his diabetes treatment. Their daily strategies remained constant throughout the fieldwork and involved administering drugs, preparing foods recommended by the doctor, weekly measurement of John's blood sugar level (using a tester kit provided by the daughter living abroad), and prayer. When the family could afford it, Diane paid for physiotherapy.

At the start of the ethnography, Diane and Hannah discussed their decision to seek ethnomedical treatment for John. They expressed frustration at the slow healing of his amputated leg and the deteriorating state of the remaining leg and fear of complications and potential amputation in the future. They needed drugs that could heal the amputated limb faster, improve the condition of the remaining leg, and prevent further complications. They chose a herbalist whose medicines, according to Hannah, had cured her aunt Patricia's husband of diabetes. All other practical routines— biomedical dietary management, prayer, and physiotherapy—would remain unchanged. They expressed great confidence in the efficacy of their chosen ethnomedical treatment and noted that in the unlikely event that this treatment failed, they would "switch back to" insulin treatment.

By the second month of fieldwork, John had received ethnomedical drugs from the herbalist. This occurred without face to face consultation. Patricia had delivered the drugs. Insulin treatment was abandoned for exclusive use of this new treatment. In addition, the family decided to consult faith healers to strengthen theefficacy of the herbal treatment. They chose a prayer camp, based in a neighbouring town, which advertised its services on radio and television and whose "miracles" had received some endorsement within their community.

AdGA: "What are your reasons for using these types of treatment?"

Hannah: "So that my dad gets healed fast."

AdGA: "Tell me some more."

Hannah: "OK, we've tried the Western type of medicine for a long time . . . but it's not getting better as we would want it; we want see the other aspect the traditional and the religious one, see whether it *will help him to be fine, even if he will be able to stand on the other foot or use the crutches since some people have been able through the religious line have been able to cure some people who are lame and who are not able to walk."*

Problems arose with the ethnomedical treatment. The drugs were ineffective. Furthermore, the herbalist had taken time off work to attend to family responsibilities, and John's family had no access for advice on treatment regimens. According to Diane, the first faith healing consultation had been positive: the principal pastor assured the family of his ability to cure John of diabetes and advised regular visits to facilitate the curative process. However, the cost of travel was high, and after two further visits to the prayer camp this mode of treatment was abandoned.

By the fourth month of fieldwork, the family had returned to exclusive use of biomedical treatment and, for adjunct spiritual support, private prayer and regular visits from Patrick. This continued for the remainder of the fieldwork. Friends and family recommended and brought a variety of herbal remedies for John's diabetes, although discussions with John and his family suggest that these remedies were not used.

[Source: de-Graft Aikins, 2005a, 2005b]

Appendix 7. Diabetes and the world of caregiving: Ruth's story

Ruth had lived with diabetes for six years. Ruth's family attributed her diabetes to a mix of diet and lifestyle factors. Although Ruth concurred with her family, she also speculated that she may have got diabetes through her brother's sorcery. She lived with severely uncontrolled diabetes and chronic physical impairments: loss of appetite, severe weight loss, joint pains, and body sores. This had a pervasive impact on her life. She was unable to carry out the simplest everyday chores and had had to abandon her previous job as a food hawker. As a result of her severe weight loss, she was labelled as having AIDS, ostracised by her community, and abandoned by her partner.

I have two close friends. But since I became sick they don't come to me anymore. ...When I sent food to the school to sell, the children wouldn't buy, because the teacher told them I have HIV/AIDS. [Ruth]

Her family became 'tainted' with the AIDS identity: they lived with 'courtesy stigma' (Goffman, 1963/1990). For example, Adjoa's attempt to take over her mother's food hawking business failed, because people were unwilling to buy food from an individual living in close proximity with an alleged AIDS sufferer.

Adjoa: *You see, at first, my mother was selling rice water ((rice pudding)). Due to her illness I had to take over and sell it but people didn't buy it anymore.*

They were thinking something different.

O: Something like what?

Adjoa: *Some people thought she had got AIDS. This perception hung over her and made people stop buying her rice water.*

In the early years, Ruth had financial support from her extended (paternal) family for biomedical treatment; but she was on insulin, which was expensive, and gradually financial support had been withdrawn. Three care givers were identified: an older daughter,

Adjoa (aged 29), widowed with three children, all of whom lived with Ruth; a son who lived locally, visited rarely, but made her annual community health insurance contributions; and a niece, Cynthia (40), a teacher, who helped financially when she could. Other forms of financial and social support came from sympathetic hospital staff and diabetes self-help group members.

Ruth's relationship with her significant others was fraught with emotionally charged misunderstandings. Misunderstandings were most acute between Ruth and Adjoa. Ruth was convinced that her family had abandoned her because they perceived her as either an AIDS sufferer or a witch.

I gave birth to twelve children, but there are only nine left. [. . .]. Those that are with me here are not responsible for my living. When they cook they don't even give me some to eat. They claim I am a witch. As a result they don't even give me food to eat. [Ruth]

Contrary to Ruth's convictions, Adjoa did not refer to her mother either as an AIDS sufferer or a witch. The family had initially believed and feared community rumours that Ruth had AIDS – her partner abandoned her as a result – but their fear had dissipated when her diabetes status was confirmed. None of Ruth's caregivers referred to her as a witch. Adjoa did not cook regularly for her mother, because she could not afford to feed her entire family regularly.

Well, I actually don't have enough money, so what I do for her is that, after selling my wares, I then go to the market to buy foodstuff and come home to cook some meal for all of us to eat. This is what I am able to do. If I have, I give her. If I don't have too, I make her aware that I don't have it. [Adjoa]

Adjoa did experience and project conflicting emotional responses onto her mother's condition. But these were underpinned by a dual struggle to cope with her own life circumstances (low income, self-employed single parent with three children) and attend to the extra daily burden brought on by her mother's physical disability and dependency. Even as Adjoa recognized the extent of her mother's impairments, she glossed over her disabilities. She criticized Ruth's inability to carry out her duties as a grandmother (e.g. taking on baby-sitting duties) and her culturally inappropriate response to her condition (emotional disintegration rather than stoicism at misfortune).

Thus, on the one hand, Adjoa stressed her intention to provide support, and on the other hand, she hoped for – and sometimes prayed for –an end to her mother's suffering, either through a miracle cure or death, to ease the emotional burden she lived with.

I am under pressure. I have realized that, in Nkoranza, if you have no one to help you in times of trouble, you worry a lot. Sometimes, I even want to travel out of town. [. . .] [. . .] when the impact of the disease increases, I feel a lot of pressure.

She worries me a lot and so I make up my mind to travel and leave her, if we leave and later we hear that she is dead, then we can come back and bury her. But I have second thoughts and then decide to stay and take care of her. [Adjoa]

In the past, Ruth had engaged with biomedical care, sporadically, when she received money from well-wishers or had treatment costs waived by sympathetic doctors at St Theresa's. During fieldwork, Ruth was predominantly medically inactive. She was hospitalized once, due to complications: hospital costs were covered by her insurance. She had no money to buy food and ate when she received donations from community members and friends. She took—often unsafe— herbal tonics to regain physical strength. She prayed and attended church regularly for spiritual support. She also attended self-help group meetings for advice and support. Self-help group members noted that while they all faced varying forms of physical disruption, Ruth experienced a particularly heavy social psychological burden.

People were saying it was AIDS because she was growing lean. She used to cook and sell maize porridge. When she sent it to the school, the children would not buy it because a teacher had told them that she was suffering from AIDS. If you are not careful, you will take poison and die. [. . .] So you see how I have grown lean? She was also a big woman. We all have problems but hers is worse.

In the past, Ruth had engaged with biomedical care, sporadically, when she received money from well-wishers or had treatment costs waived by sympathetic doctors at St Theresa's. During fieldwork, Ruth was predominantly medically inactive. She was hospitalized once, due to complications: hospital costs were covered by her insurance. She had no money to buy food and ate when she received donations from community members and friends. She took—often unsafe—herbal tonics to regain physical strength. She prayed and attended church regularly for spiritual support. She also attended self-help group meetings for advice and support. Self-help group members noted that while they all faced varying forms of physical disruption, Ruth experienced a particularly heavy social psychological burden.

People were saying it was AIDS because she was growing lean. She used to cook and sell maize porridge. When she sent it to the school, the children would not buy it because a teacher had told them that she was suffering from AIDS. If you are not careful, you will take poison and die. [. . .] So you see how I have grown lean? She was also a big woman. We all have problems but hers is worse.

[Jane, self-help group member]

Ruth's interview narratives were dominated by despair at the extent and severity of the impact of diabetes to her life. She frequently cried during interviews. She prayed for death to end to her chronic suffering. However, even as she was repeatedly drawn to suicide, she noted she was unable to go through with such a course of action, because her Christian faith abhorred suicide as a response to life's misfortunes.

Recently, I even thought of committing suicide by poisoning myself. [. . .] [. . .] And I say

it each day. But I remind myself later on that, it is the Lord who brought me into this world. And if I make my mind up about poisoning myself there would be a punishment for me one day. But I think of it very much. [Ruth]

[Source: de-Graft Aikins, 2005a, 2005b, 2006]

Appendix 8. Hope for a cure: a driver for healershopping

For many Ghanaians with diabetes, enduring diabetes is the dominant emotional response, as is hope for the end to diabetes. Many, therefore, hover between endurance and hope. For the most part, endurance enforces a commitment to biomedical management. During moments of vulnerability – physical, psychological, spiritual - hope became a powerful force, leading to experimentation with cures. These moments are experienced by almost everyone, including educated wealthy urban individuals such as Opanin, who by their own accounts ought to know better.

"And I'll tell you a story. Just about a week and a half ago, a chap came and sold me a traditional thing. He was so excited convincing me of the efficacy of this thing. So I said, "my friend the diabetes does not care about these things and as far as I know, it's a pancreas dysfunctional problem so how're you going to 'tu asee' (remove, cure)". And he was like "oh, I'm telling you the pancreas will work and blah blah blah", and I said "ok". I couldn't see how this thing will repair a broken down pancreas anyway, but he was so persuasive, so aggressive, so I said all right, I'll try it. I took it. The trouble with the herbalist.... dosages is all a big act of faith. But the chap told me [he was working with] a chap trained from America and so on and so forth and was very convincing in the efficiency of the drug. So I said "ok". So they came with a gallon full of preparation or concoction, whatever it was and I took it. And my first testing was dramatic y'know...but I think I had a bit of diarrhoe, a real retch, then the second day (and he was telling me to drink it like water, you won't take water, you're supposed to take this)[...AdGA: This as a substitute for water...]

So I took in a little more on the second day, and Christ Jesus!, it looked as if there was acid in the thing, it was really eating in my stomach, really. I couldn't sleep, I went to the toilet and nothing and nothing was coming but this thing...I was retching, so the next day, I decided that I wouldn't take any. Then everybody started laughing y'know. If you went to the doctor and the doctor started asking you, why you took it, and did you know what you were taking, what would you say? And I came round to saying that this is all very stupid so I stopped it."

[Source: de-Graft Aikins, 2005b]

Appendix 9. NCD prevention and control responses from selected low and middle income countries

(Source: de-Graft Aikins and Agyemang, 2017)

Strengthening health systems for NCD prevention and control: best practice responses and interventions

Concepts and strategies for strengthening health systems basic building blocks	Practical responses and interventions in selected LMICs
Service delivery Integrated care models (integrating healthcare models that address multiple health service needs, usually at the primary care level) Diagonal approach to health service delivery (a synthesis of the vertical approach[disease-specific intervention on a mass scale]and horizontal approach [integrated resource-sharing health service])	In Cambodia, Ethiopia, Malawi, Thailand and Vietnam, HIV/AIDS programmes have been used as a platform for providing NCD (including diabetes and hypertension) care In South Africa and Uganda, integrated care models used for treating co-morbid physical and mental health conditions with significant improvements in health outcomes

Concepts and strategies for strengthening health systems basic building blocks	Practical responses and interventions in selected LMICs
Health workforce Task shifting *(rational distribution of tasks among health workforce teams, involving shifting healthcare tasks from higher-trained health workers to less skilled health workers)*	In rural Cameroon and rural Iran non-physician clinicians and community health workers, respectively, trained to provide diabetes and hypertension care. Ghana pilot CVD interventions in urban poor communities involve community health workers from the urban Community-based Health Planning and Services (CHPS) programme In Haiti, Rwanda and Uganda, nurses are trained to deliver chemotherapy for cancer (palliative) care In India, Pakistan, Uganda and Zimbabwe community health workers are trained to provide interventions for depression
Medicines and technology Advocating for access to cheap and safe medicines and technologies	The African Organization for Research and Training in Cancer (AORTIC) lobbies African governments to cut taxes on cancer drugs and medical equipment In Cameroon a multi-institutional partnership led to improved access to affordable diabetes medicines and technologies

Concepts and strategies for strengthening health systems basic building blocks	Practical responses and interventions in selected LMICs
Information systems NCD surveillance	LMIC focused NCD surveillance initiatives include the WHO STEPwise approach to risk factor Surveillance (STEPS) and the WHO STEPwise approach to stroke surveillance (STEPS Stroke), the Global Tobacco Surveillance System (GTSS), the International Network for the Demographic Evaluation of Populations and Their Health (INDEPTH Network), the WHO Study on global AGEing and adult Health (SAGE). ················ China, India and Pakistan have developed national and sub-regional surveillance initiatives for diabetes and CVD.
Financing Social insurance; Social franchising *(a network of private providers providing a common brand of products and services)*	Rwanda: HIV funding programmes used to expand health insurance coverage for poor people living with multiple conditions including NCDs . ················ In Colombia, Mexico, Pakistan and Thailand social insurance schemes including NCDs are provided. ················ In Bangladesh, the NGO Health Service Delivery Programme funded by USAID provides integrated services for maternal and child health, infectious diseases and selected NCDs.

Concepts and strategies for strengthening health systems basic building blocks	Practical responses and interventions in selected LMICs
Leadership and governance Political investment in population-based interventions; Operationalising 'multifaceted, multi-institutional frameworks' and the 'whole of government, whole of society approach' to NCD prevention , control and advocacy	In Brazil, China, India, Indonesia, Mauritius and South Africa, governments and state agencies have instituted a NCD intervention programmes at city or national levels using the 'multi-faceted, multi-institutional' framework. These projects have led to reductions in target NCD risk factors as well as morbidity and mortality rates In Bangladesh, Ethiopia, India, Rwanda and Thailand, favourable health outcomes have been attributed to good governance and political commitment. Initiatives include making drugs accessible and affordable and leveraging development assistance to expand health workforce and infrastructure with knock on effects on NCD care . In Africa, the Mental Health and Poverty Project (MHaPP) and Mental Health Leadership and Advocacy programme (mhLAP) aim to improve mental health care in 8 countries: Gambia, Ghana, Liberia, Nigeria, Sierra Leone, South Africa, Uganda, Zambia. Rwanda spearheads the NCD Synergies movement to improve NCD care for the poorest in Africa and LMICs.

Concepts and strategies for strengthening health systems basic building blocks	Practical responses and interventions in selected LMICs
People (as health systems recipients and producers) Healthcare/care/help seeking; Self-help; Education; Empowerment; Participation	Community-based CVD interventions in Argentina, Brazil, Cambodia, Cameroon, China, Ghana, India, Indonesia, Iran, Mauritius, Mexico, Pakistan, South Africa, Turkey, Vietnam employ a mix of didactic, mass mediated and participatory approaches to education and risk reduction. .... NCD self-help and advocacy groups include: cancer groups in Brazil, China, Ghana, India, Kenya, Malaysia, and Pakistan [44]; mental health groups in Ghana, Kenya, Rwanda, South Africa, Tanzania and Zambia [45]; aged support in Egypt and Thailand. These groups provide health and disease specific education, social support and improved psychological and health outcomes. .... The NCD Alliance has created a platform for a global network of over 2000 NCD civil society groups from 170 countries (including LMICs) placed under 7 categories: federation member associations; NGOs; academic institutions; research institutes; patient support organizations; scientific associations and professional societies.

REFERENCES

Abubakari AR, Lauder W, Agyemang C et al. (2008). Prevalence and time trends in obesity among adult West African populations : a meta-analysis. *Obesity Reviews*. 9:297–311.

Addo, J., Agyemang, C., Smeeth, L., de-Graft Aikins, A., Edusei, A.K., Ogedegbe, O. (2012). A review of population-based studies on hypertension in Ghana. *Ghana Medical Journal*, 46 (2), 4-11.

Agyei-Mensah, S. and de-Graft Aikins, A. (2010). Epidemiological transition and the double burden of disease in Accra, Ghana. *Journal of Urban Health, 87 (5), 879–897.*

Agyemang, C., Addo, J., Bhopal, R., de-Graft Aikins, A., and Stronks, K. (2009). Cardiovascular disease, diabetes and established risks factors among populations of sub-Saharan African descent in Europe: a literature review. *Globalization and Health*, 5: 7.

Agyemang, C., Buene, E.A., Meeks, K., Owusu-Dabo, E., de-Graft Aikins, A, et al. (2014) Research on Obesity and Type 2 Diabetes among African Migrants: The RODAM study. *BMJ Open*.4:e004877. doi:10.1136/bmjopen-2014-004877.

Agyemang, C, Meeks, K. Beune, E., Owusu-Dabo, E., Mockenhaupt, F., Addo, J., de-Graft Aikins, A., Bahendeka, S., Danquah, I., Schulze, M., Spranger, J., Burr, T.; Adjei Baffour, P.; Amoah, A., Galbete, C., Henneman, P.; Klipstein-Grobusch, K., Nicolaou, M.; Adeyemo, A.,; van Straalen; J., Smeeth, L., Stronks, K. (2016a). Obesity and Type 2 Diabetes in Sub-Saharan Africans - Is the burden in today's Africa similar to African migrants in Europe? - The RODAM study. *BMC Medicine*, **14**:166 (**DOI:** 10.1186/s12916-016-0709-0)

Agyemang, C., Boatemaa S., Agyemang G., and de-Graft Aikins, A. (2016b) Obesity in Africa. In R. Ahima (Ed), *Metabolic syndrome: A comprehensive textbook*. Springer International Publishing, Switzerland.

Akotia, C.S. and Mate-Kole, C.C. (2014). Psychology: Readings from Ghana. Accra: DigiBooks Ghana Ltd.

Awah. P.K and Phillimore, P. (2008). Diabetes, medicine and modernity in Cameroon. *Africa* 78 (4), 475-495.

Awah, P.K, Unwin, N and Phillimore, P (2008) Cure or control: complying with biomedical regime of diabetes in Cameroon. *BMC Health Services Research, 8,43.*

Awuah, R.B., Anarfi, J.K., Agyemang, C., Ogedegbe, G. and de-Graft Aikins, A. (2014) Prevalence, awareness, treatment and control of hypertension in urban poor communities in Accra, Ghana. *Journal of Hypertension.* 32(6), 1203-10

Babor, T.F., and Higgins-Biddle, J.C. (2001). Brief Interventions for hazardous and harmful drinking. Geneva: WHO.

Bosu WK. (2012). A comprehensive review of the policy and programmatic response to rising chronic non-communicable disease in Ghana. *Ghana Medical Journal, 46(2), 69–78.*

Burton, M., and Kagan, C. (2005) Liberation Social Psychology: Learning From Latin America. *Journal of Community and Applied Social Psychology,* 15(1), 63 –78.

Bury, M. (1982). Chronic illness as biographical disruption. *Sociology of Health and Illness,* 4, 167-182.

Campbell, C. and Jovchelovitch, S. (2000). Health, Community and Development: Towards a Social Psychology of Participation. *Journal of Community & Applied Social Psychology,* 10: 255 – 270.

Campbell, R., Pound, P., Pope, C., Britten, N., Pill, R., Morgan, M., Donovan, J. (2003). Evaluating meta-ethnography: a synthesis of qualitative research on lay experiences of diabetes and diabetes care. *Social Science & Medicine,* 56, 671–684

Carel, H. (2007). Can I be ill and happy? *Philosophia,* 35:95–110

Charmaz, K. (1983). Loss of self: a fundamental form of suffering in the chronically ill. *Sociology of Health and Illness,* 5(2), 168 – 195.

Christopher, J.C., Wendt, D.C., Marecek, J., and Goodman, D.M. (2014). Critical Cultural Awareness. Contributions to a Globalizing Psychology. *American Psychologist,* 69(7), 645-655.

Clarke, J. (2014) Medicalization of global health 3: the medicalization of the non-communicable diseases agenda. *Glob Health Action,* 7: 24002

Crossley, M. (2000). *Rethinking Health Psychology.* Buckingham: Open University Press.

Dedey F, Wu L., Ayettey AH, Sanuade OA, Akingbola TS, Hewlett SA, Tayo BO, Cole H, de-Graft Aikins A, Ogedegbe G, Adanu R. (2016). Factors associated with waiting time for Breast Cancer treatment in a Teaching Hospital in Ghana. *Health Education and Behaviour*, 1-8, DOI: 10.1177/1090198115620417

de-Graft Aikins, A. (2003). Living with diabetes in rural and urban Ghana: a critical social psychological examination of illness action and scope for intervention. *Journal of Health Psychology*, 8(5), 557-72

de-Graft Aikins, A. (2004). Strengthening quality and continuity of diabetes care in rural Ghana: a critical social psychological approach. *Journal of Health Psychology*, 2004, 9(2), 295-309.

de-Graft Aikins, A. (2005a). Healer-shopping in Africa: new evidence from a rural-urban qualitative study of Ghanaian diabetes experiences. *British Medical Journal*, 331, 737.

de-Graft Aikins, A. (2005b). *Social representations of diabetes in Ghana: reconstructing self, society and culture.* Unpublished PhD Thesis, London School of Economics and Political Science.

de-Graft Aikins, A. (2006). Reframing applied disease stigma research: a multilevel analysis of diabetes stigma in Ghana. *Journal of Community and Applied Social Psychology*, 16(6), 426-441.

de-Graft Aikins, A. (2012). Familiarising the unfamiliar: cognitive polyphasia, emotions and the creation of social representations. *Papers on Social Representations*, 21, 7.1-7.28.

de-Graft Aikins, A. (2014). Social cognition, social representations and social knowledge: themes in Ghanaian social psychology. In C. Mate-Kole and C Akotia (Eds), Psychology: Readings from Ghana. Accra: DigiBooks Ghana Ltd. (pages 249-272)

de-Graft Aikins, A. (2015). Mental illness and destitution in Ghana: a social psychological perspective. In Emmanuel Akyeampong, Alan Hill and Arthur Kleinman. (Eds). *The Culture of Mental Illness and Psychiatric Practice in Africa*. Bloomington: Indiana University Press. (pages 112-143)

de-Graft Aikins, A. & Ofori-Atta, A. (2007) Homelessness and mental health in Ghana: everyday experiences of Accra's migrant squatters. *Journal of Health Psychology, 12(5)*, 761-778.

de-Graft Aikins, A. and Marks, D.F. (2007). Health, disease and healthcare in Africa *Journal of Health Psychology*, 12(3). 387-402

de-Graft Aikins, A., Unwin, N., Agyemang, C. Allotey, P., Campbell, C and Arhinful, D.K. (2010). Tackling Africa's Chronic Disease Burden: from the local to the global. *Globalization and Health*, 6:5.

de-Graft Aikins, A., Boynton, P. and Atanga, L.L. (2010) Developing Effective Chronic Disease Prevention in Africa: insights from Ghana and Cameroon. *Globalization and Health*, 6:6.

de-Graft Aikins, A, Pitchforth, E., Allotey, P., Ogedegbe, G., Agyemang, C. (2012). Culture, ethnicity and chronic conditions: reframing concepts and methods for research, intervention and policy in low and middle income countries. *Ethnicity & Health*, 17(6), 551-561.

de-Graft Aikins, A., Anum, A., Agyemang, C., Addo, J. and Ogedegbe, O. (2012). Lay representations of chronic diseases in Ghana: implications for primary prevention. *Ghana Medical Journal*, 46(2), 59-68.

de-Graft Aikins, A., Agyei-Mensah, S., Agyemang, C. (Eds). (2013) Ghana's Chronic Non-communicable disease burden: multidisciplinary perspectives. Accra: Sub Saharan Publishers

de-Graft Aikins, A., Awuah, R.B., Pera T., Mendez, M., Ogedegbe, G (2014a). Explanatory models of diabetes in poor urban Ghanaian communities. *Ethnicity and Health*. Jul 22: 1-18 (DOI: 10.1080/13557858.2014.921896)

de-Graft Aikins, A., Kushitor, M., Koram, K., Gyamfi, S., Ogedegbe. G. (2014b). Chronic non-communicable diseases and the challenge of universal health coverage. Insights from community-based cardiovascular disease research in urban poor communities in Accra, Ghana. *BMC Public Health*. 14 (Suppl 2).

de-Graft Aikins, A., Ofori-Atta A., Anum, A., Dzokoto, V. (2014c) Psychology in Ghana: a review of research and practice. In S. Agyei-Mensah, A. Oduro and J. Ayee (Eds) Changing Perspectives in the Social Sciences in Ghana. Dordrecht: Springer. (pages 75-93)

de-Graft Aikins, A., Dzokoto, V., Yevak, E. (2015) Mass media constructions of 'socio-psychological epidemics' in sub-Saharan Africa: the case of genital shrinking in 11 countries. *Public Understanding of Science. 24: 988-1006,*

de-Graft Aikins, A. and Agyemang, C. (Eds) (2016). *Chronic non-communicable diseases in low and middle income countries.* Oxon: CABI Publishers.

de-Graft Aikins, A., and Agyemang, C. (2017). Chronic non-communicable diseases in low and middle income countries: concepts and strategies for prevention, control and advocacy. *CAB Reviews, 12 (027),* doi10.1079/PAVSNNR201712027.

de-Graft Aikins, A. and Koram, K. (2017). Health and Healthcare Financing in Ghana, 1957-2017. In E. Aryeetey and R. Kanbur (Eds). *The Economy of Ghana: Sixty Years after Independence.* Oxford: Oxford University Press.

Doise, W. (1986). *Levels of explanation in social psychology.* Cambridge: Cambridge University Press.

Faircloth, C.A., Boylstein, C., Rittman, M., Young, M.E. Gubrium, J. (2004). Sudden illness and biographical flow in narratives of stroke recovery. *Sociology of Health and Illness,* 26(2), 242-261.

Feierman, S., & Janzen, J. M. (Eds.) (1992). *The social basis of health and healing in Africa.* Berkeley: University of California Press.

Field, M.J. (1937). *Religion and medicine of the Ga people.* Oxford University Press.

Gervais, M., Morant, N., & Penn, G. (1999). Making sense of "absence": Towards a typology of absence in social representations theory and research. *Journal for the Theory of Social Behaviour, 29* (4), 419-444.

Goffman, E. (1963/1990). Stigma: Notes on the management of spoiled identity. New Jersey: Prentice-Hall.

Goody, J. (Ed.) (1975). *Changing social structure in Ghana: Essays in the comparative sociology of a new state and an old tradition.* London: International African Institute.

Helman, C. (2000). *Culture, health and illness.* Oxford; Boston: Butterworth-Heineman.

Hepworth, J. (2004). Public health psychology: A conceptual and practical framework. *Journal of Health Psychology* 2004, 9(1):41-54.

Janzen, J. (with Arkinstall, W.) (1982). *The quest for therapy in Lower Zaire.* Berkeley: University of California Press.

Katz, A.H. (1981). Self-help and mutual aid: an emerging social movement? *Annual Review of Sociology* 7, 129–155.

Kleinman, A. (1980). *Patients and Healers in the Context of Culture: An exploration of the borderland between Anthropology, Medicine, and Psychiatry.* California: University of California Press.

Kolling M, Winkley K, von Deden M (2010). "For someone who's rich, it's not a problem". Insights from Tanzania on diabetes health-seeking and medical pluralism among Dar es Salaam's urban poor. *Globalization and Health, 6:8.*

Kuhn, T. (1962). *The structure of scientific revolutions.* Chicago : University of Chicago Press.

Last, M. (1992). The importance of knowing about not knowing: Observations from Hausaland. In S. Feierman & J.M. Janzen (Eds), *The Social Basis of Health and Healing in Africa.* Berkeley: University of California Press. Pp 393-406.

Lightfoot, C.S. (2003). Expert patients usher in a new era of opportunity for the NHS. *British Medical Journal,* 326.

Markova, I., & Farr, R. (1995). *Representations of health, illness and handicap.* UK: Harwood.

McCool, A. (2015). "African electronics" takes a spiritual approach to individual power. (https://creators.vice.com)

Mendis, S and Chestnov, O. (2016). The global response for prevention and control of chronic non-communicable diseases: key milestones and outcomes. In A. de-Graft Aikins and C. Agyemang, (Eds). *Chronic non-communicable diseases in low and middle income countries.* Oxon: CABI Publishers. (pp.194-208)

Moscovici, S and Duveen, G (2001). *Social representations: Explorations in Social Psychology.* New York: New York University Press.

Moscovici, S and Markova, I. (2006). *The Making of Modern Social Psychology. The hidden story of how an International Social Science was Created.* Cambridge: Polity Press.

Moscovici, S. (2008). *Psychoanalysis. Its Image and Its Public.* Cambridge: Polity Press.

Moscovici, S. (1998). Social consciousness and its history. *Culture and Psychology*, 4(3), 411- 429.

Mullings, L. (1984). *Therapy, Ideology and Social Change: Mental Healing in Urban Ghana.* Berkeley: University of California Press.

Murray, M. (2000). Levels of Narrative analysis in health Psychology. *Journal of Health Psychology*, 5(3) 337–347.

Paterson, B., Thorne, S., Dewis, M. (1998). Adapting to and Managing Diabetes. *Image: Journal of Nursing Scholarship*, 30(1), 57-62.

Quayson, A. (2014). *Oxford Street, Accra. City Life and the itineraries of Transnationalism.* Durham and London: Duke University Press

Radley, A. (1994). *Making sense of illness.* London: Sage.

Reeve, J., Lloyd-Williams, M., Payne, S. And Dowrick, C. (2010). Revisiting biographical disruption: Exploring individual embodied illness experience in people with terminal cancer. *Health*, 14(2): 178–195.

Rekdal, O. B. (1999). Cross-cultural healing in east African ethnography. *Medical Anthropology Quarterly*, 13(4), 458-82

Richards, G. (1997). *'Race', Racism and Psychology. Towards a reflexive history.* London: Routledge.

Robertson, C., (1984). *Sharing the same bowl: a socioeconomic history of women and class in Accra, Ghana.* Bloomington: Indiana University Press.

Rose D., Efraim D, Gervais M, Joffe H, Jovchelovitch S, Morant N. Questioning consensus in social representations theory. *Papers on Social Representations* 1995;4(2):1–155.

Ryan, G.W. (1998). What do sequential behavioural patterns suggest about the medical decision-making process? Modeling home case management of acute illness in a rural Cameroonian village. *Social Science and Medicine*, 46 (2): 209-25.

Sackrey, C., Schneider, G., and Knoedler, J. (2013). Introduction to political economy. Boston: Economic Affairs Bureau Inc. *Research (IDR) Reports*, 11(6), 1-21.

Scheper-Hughes, N. and Lock, M. (1987). The Mindful Body: A Prolegomenon to Future Work in Medical Anthropology. *Medical Anthropology Quarterly*, 1(1), 6-41.

Strahl, H. (2003). Cultural interpretations of an emerging health problem: blood pressure in Dar es Salaam, Tanzania. *Anthropology & Medicine, 10 (3), 309-324.*

Suhrcke M, Nugent RA, Stuckler D, Rocco L (2006). *Chronic Disease: An Economic Perspective* London: Oxford Health Alliance; 2006.

Van der Geest, S. (2004). Dying peacefully: Considering good death and bad death in Kwahu-Tafo, Ghana. *Social Science & Medicine,* 58 (5): 899-912.

WHO (2005). *Preventing Chronic Disease. A vital investment* Geneva: WHO.

Professor Ama de-Graft Aikins: a Profile

Ama de-Graft Aikins is Professor of Social Psychology at the Regional Institute for Population Studies (RIPS), and Dean of International Programmes, University of Ghana (UG). She has a BSc (Hons) in Pharmacology from the University of Manchester (1994) and an MSc in Psychological Studies from Manchester Metropolitan University (1998). She received her PhD in Social Psychology from the London School of Economics and Political Science (LSE) in 2005 and completed postdoctoral training at the University of Cambridge in 2006. After research and teaching positions at the University of Cambridge and LSE, she joined UG as a senior lecturer in October 2009. She was promoted to Associate Professor in October 2011 and to full professor in February 2015. She is the first female full professor of psychology at the University of Ghana.

Ama de-Graft Aikins' research focuses primarily on experiences and representations of chronic physical and mental illnesses, Africa's chronic non-communicable disease (NCD) burden, and the social psychology of knowledge production in African settings. With an undergraduate background in pharmacology and training in the critical social psychology tradition at master's and doctoral levels, her work is informed by interdisciplinarity. She has actively sought mentorship and collaboration from academics in the medical and health sciences, social sciences and humanities. She has conducted independent research as well as collaborative research based in Ghana, Europe and the US with colleagues from the University of Ghana, University of Amsterdam, New York University (NYU) and London School of Hygiene and Tropical Medicine (LSHTM).

Ama de-Graft Aikins' independent and collaborative research has attracted competitive grants and commissioned funds from major funders, including the Economic and Social Research Council

(ESRC), the British Academy (BA), the European Union, Grand Challenges Canada and the World Health Organization (WHO). Her research has produced over 100 peer-reviewed scholarly publications, including 10 edited volumes. She has presented her research at over 100 conferences, high level meetings and university seminars in 25 countries. She is involved in NCD advocacy and health systems and policy research and has consulted for institutions including the Ghana Health Service (GHS) and WHO. Her NCD research has attracted international media attention including features in the UK Guardian and The Economist.

Ama de-Graft Aikins has taught undergraduate and graduate courses at the LSE, Cambridge and UG. She has supervised over 40 masters theses in Social Psychology, Social Policy, Public Health and Population Studies at UG, LSE, LSHTM, NYU and the University of Sussex. She has supervised 10 PhD students in Population Studies and Public Health at UG, University of Amsterdam and Australian Catholic University. She has contributed to the development of models for training graduate students and early career researchers in the social sciences and humanities in Africa through her association with BA, the Association of Commonwealth Universities (ACU), the African Studies Association, UK (ASAUK) and the LSE African Initiative.

Ama de-Graft Aikins has received prestigious awards and fellowships, including The Economic and Social Research Council (ESRC) postdoctoral fellowship (2005), Aspen Ideas Festival Scholar award (2009), Inter-Academy Panel (IAP) Outstanding Young Scientist award (2011) and the LSE African Initiative Fellowship (2013). She is a visiting senior fellow at the LSE and University College London, and a fellow of the Ghana Academy of Arts and Sciences.

INDEX

Printed in the United States
By Bookmasters